LANGUAGE DISTURBANCE AND INTELLECTUAL FUNCTIONING

JANUA LINGUARUM

STUDIA MEMORIAE
NICOLAI VAN WIJK DEDICATA

edenda curat

C. H. VAN SCHOONEVELD

INDIANA UNIVERSITY

SERIES MINOR

NR. 48

1969
MOUTON
THE HAGUE · PARIS

LANGUAGE DISTURBANCE AND INTELLECTUAL FUNCTIONING

A COMPARISON OF THE PERFORMANCES OF HEMIPLEGIC PATIENTS WITH APHASIA AND HEMIPLEGIC PATIENTS WITHOUT APHASIA IN NON-VERBAL TASKS OF INTELLECTUAL FUNCTIONING

by

CARL KENNETH LUBIN

1969
MOUTON
THE HAGUE · PARIS

LIBRARY OF CONGRESS CATALOG CARD NUMBER 68-17904

Printed in The Netherlands by Mouton & Co., Printers, The Hague.

ACKNOWLEDGEMENTS

An endeavor such as this requires the cooperation, assistance and encouragement of many. It is difficult fully to express the gratitude the writer feels toward his friends and colleagues for their efforts during the course of this study.

To the late Professor Brian Tomlinson whose patient guidance and critical analysis contributed much to the final form of this work, the writer is greatly indebted. The writer will remember always the effort, kindness and encouragement of Professors Elizabeth Addoms and Edward Kemp.

For making available the facilities and subjects for this study, the writer is obligated to Dr. Milton Lowenthal of the Bird S. Coler Hospital and Home and to Dr. Aaron Weiss of the Bellevue Hospital Rehabilitation Service. Appreciation is expressed to the staffs of these installations for their cooperation as it is to Dr. Leonard Diller of the Institute of Physical Medicine and Rehabilitation for his advice. Thanks are extended to Mr. Robert Reichard for his cooperation and advice on matters statistical and to Mrs. Susan Jacobson for her careful editing.

Finally, sincere gratitude is expressed to my wife whose secretarial efforts, patience and understanding contributed much to the final conclusion of this research.

C. K. L.

TABLE OF CONTENTS

LIST OF TABLES

INTRODUCTION

"None of the theories of the various types of aphasia have had general acceptance. Despite a century of study, the mechanisms of speech and aphasia remain as challenging problems."[1]

Although the literature in the areas of brain organization and functioning, as well as the relationship between brain damage and intelligence, or between language and thought, is more than substantial, the entire field is still a scientific frontier. There is as much disagreement as agreement among the authorities in all these areas.

The end of World War II saw significant strides made in the field of rehabilitation, with numerous installations established in the United States and many other nations around the world. The demands of the war brought into focus the need for the rehabilitation of the disabled. Granick states:

The Second World War has left us with a substantial group of aphasic patients. If we approach these men as cases for retraining and positive rehabilitation, we may expect also that the extended process of retraining, properly carried out, will turn up a wealth of insight into the nature of brain functioning, the primary mental abilities, and the general reactions of the brain injured.[2]

Subsequent military engagements increased the population of brain-damaged and aphasic individuals. Traffic and industrial accidents are daily adding to the number of brain-damaged persons in all age groups.

As the average life expectancy increases, there has been a concomitant increase in the number of people suffering *strokes*. It has been estimated that there are approximately one million hemi-

[1] W. Penfield and L. Roberts, *Speech and Brain Mechanisms*, p. 81.
[2] Louis Granick, *Aphasia, A Guide to Retraining*, p. 11.

plegics in the United States, and that one-third of these are aphasic to some degree.[3]

With the improved medical and surgical techniques many of these are surviving who in the past might have died. Wepman as well as others believe that many of these patients can be rehabilitated and enabled to "lead much more useful and satisfying lives than now seem possible for them."[4]

However, in a rehabilitation program, the ability and capacity of the patient for learning and retraining is crucial. To what extent does the loss of language interfere with the intellectual functioning of the aphasic? After being in the field of rehabilitation for several years, this study was undertaken because it was believed that it would contribute additional information to the existing body of knowledge, not only in the field of rehabilitation, but to theory in the areas of the organization and functioning of the brain. Hopefully, it would make for a better understanding of the relationship of language to intellectual functioning, as well as the relationship of intellectual functioning to brain damage. It would open up also further possibilities for research in these important areas.

Briefly, this book is divided into six chapters. In the first chapter, a summary of reported research and literature pertinent to the current investigation, is given. Chapter 2 presents the problem, delimitations, assumption, and hypothesis of the study. This is followed in Chapter 3 by a description of the research setting and populations as well as the evaluative devices employed, while Chapter 4 describes how the data was treated. The fifth chapter discusses the results of the study, and the final chapter presents a summary and conclusions based on the study and recommendations.

[3] "Rehabilitation of the Hemiplegic", pp. 5-19.
[4] J. M. Wepman, *Recovery from Aphasia*, p. 7.

1. RELATED LITERATURE

Since comprehensive reviews of this literature have been made by others,[1] this chapter will present only a summary of the diverse opinions in the various areas with which this study is concerned. Included in this review are: 1) concepts of brain organization and function; 2) the relationship of brain damage to intelligence; 3) the relationship of language to thought; 4) the question of the lateralization of cerebral function.

BRAIN ORGANIZATION AND FUNCTION

From ancient times, the idea has persisted that different parts of the brain perform different functions. "The Hippocratic treatise on head injuries noted that wounds of the temporal region on one side might result in convulsions on the opposite side of the body."[2] There were many such observations throughout the following centuries, but they did not lead to the development of any over-all theory. However, they may have laid the groundwork for the more recent developments of the 19th century.

Nineteenth Century Researchers

Gall, at the turn of the 19th century, stated the doctrine of cerebral localization. Emphasizing dissection rather than section as a method of investigation of the brain, he concluded that "the convolutions of the brain must be recognized as the parts where the instincts,

[1] H. Head (1926), Weisenberg and McBride (1935), B. Blatt (1949), H. Chenven (1953), Penfield and Roberts (1959). A biliography on aphasia is presented by R. R. Leutenagger (1953), Wepman, J. M. (1961).

[2] Harry Helson, *Theoretical Foundations of Psychology*, p. 87.

sentiments, penchants, talents, and in general, the moral and intellectual forces are exercised."[3] He believed that the memory for words was located in the frontal lobes of the brain. Normal speech, for Gall, was due to the perfect exercise of certain aspects of memory each of which was situated in some particular part of the anterior lobes of the brain. In this work he was aided by Spurzheim, a student of his, who in 1815 separated from him and adopted the term *phrenology* from a Dr. Thomas Foster. Spurzheim wrote many independent works, and lectured widely in England, Europe, and the U.S.A.[4] Flourens (1823) attempted to contravert the doctrine of localization and postulated that "all parts of the brain served the same function of any other portion in case of injury or disease."[5] Bouillaud, in 1825, questioned Flourens' concept and localized the organs of articulate speech in the anterior lobes of the brain. "In particular, the movements of the organs of speech are regulated by a special cerebral center, distinct and independent. This is situated in the anterior lobes of the brain."[6]

In 1861, Broca[7] went far beyond all predecessors, by localizing a center for *articulated language* in the posterior portion of the left third frontal convolution. This observation was based on *aphemics*, in whose brains circumscribed lesions were evident at autopsy.

Soon after Broca presented his findings, Charcot and Trousseau reported cases of aphemia. Trousseau took exception to the term aphemia, claiming the Greek meaning of the word at that time was *infamy*. He substituted the term aphasia, which became the accepted term. The neurological dispute moved to England where in 1867, Ogle introduced the term *agraphia*. Bastian believed that one thought with words and that there were different specific centers with fiber connections, the most important of which was the auditory word center. He stated that the destruction of Broca's area produced loss of kinesthetic memory. In his writings on aphasia

[3] *Ibid.*, p. 88.

[4] Gordon W. Allport, *Personality: A Psychological Interpretation*, p. 79.

[5] J. M. Nielson, *Agnosis, Apraxia, Aphasia*, p. 1.

[6] H. Head, *Aphasia and Kindred Disorders of Speech*, p. 16.

[7] P. Broca, "A Translation of Broca's Original Article on the Location of the Speech Center", pp. 16-20, translated by J. Kann.

which started in 1869 and lasted for about thirty years, he was the first to describe *word deafness and word blindness.*

Jackson made significant contributions to the understanding of aphasia. He was the first to describe partial imperception, as well as apraxia of the tongue. He reported the first case of a left-handed man with a lesion of the right hemisphere and aphasia.

Jackson took issue with the advocates of localization.

> Whilst I believe that the hinder part of the left third frontal convolution is the part most often damaged, I do not localize speech in any such small part of the brain. To locate the damage which destroys speech and to locate speech are two different things.[8]

He believed the whole brain was involved in speech.

> To coin the word verbalizing to include all the ways in which words serve, I would assert that both halves of the brain are alike in that each serve in verbalizing.[9]

By this, he did not mean that the two halves of the brain are double or such exact duplicates that either half will do for speech because he realized that it was a matter of most significance that damage to but one hemisphere would make a man speechless.

It was his opinion that:

> Perceptions (concepts, images, perception, etc.) develop words automatically in no order, or rather in their own order, on the right side of the brain. Words are, or may be objectively considered on the left, put into new relations, made into propositions. The links between these two revivals are, I imagine, the perceptions of which the words are arbitrary signs.[10]

This dual functioning of the brain, according to Jackson, explained why the aphasic lost propositional speech but might retain emotional speech, recurrent utterances and jargon. He distinguishes between these two aspects of language and states:

> To speak is not simply to utter words, it is to propositionize. A proposition is such a relation of words that it makes one new meaning; not by a mere addition of what we call the separate meanings of the several words;

[8] Henry Head, *op. cit.*, p. 81.
[9] W. Penfield and L. Roberts, *op. cit.*, p. 62.
[10] W. Penfield and L. Roberts, *op. cit.*, p. 89.

... Single words are meaningless, and so is any unrelated succession of words. The unit of speech is a proposition.[11]

He continued:

Loss of speech is therefore the loss of power to propositionize. It is not only the power to propositionize aloud (to talk), but to propositionize either internally or externally, and it may exist when the patient remains able to mutter some words.[12]

After studying seventy-two of his own patients and analyzing all the extant theories of localization, Bateman concluded:

That although something may be said in favor of each of the popular theories of the localization of speech, still, so many exceptions to each of them have been recorded that they will none of them bear the test of a disinterested and impartial scrutiny.[13]

He goes on to say:

That I by no means consider it proved that there is a cerebral center for speech at all, and I would venture to suggest that speech, like the soul, may be something the comprehension of which is beyond the limits of our finite minds.[14]

Echoes of the controversy came from Germany where Fritsch and Hitzig in 1870 demonstrated that electrical stimulation of the frontal cortex in the dog and other mammals resulted in movements of the extremity of the opposite side. In 1874, Hitzig delimited even more accurately the motor area of the dog and monkey. Ferrier, in 1873, showed that removal of the *hand area* in the brain of the monkey resulted in a paralysis of the opposite hand.

Wernicke,[15] 1874, isolated an auditory speech area which he located in the first temporal convolution. A lesion in this area, he found, produced a loss of understanding of speech. He believed that the anterior half of the brain was concerned with the concept of movement and the posterior (including the temporal lobe) with

[11] J. Hughling Jackson, *Selected Writings of J. Hughling Jackson*, pp. 159-160.
[12] *Loc. cit.*
[13] Frederic Bateman, *On Aphasia or Loss of Speech and the Localization of the Faculty of Articulate Language*, p. 212.
[14] Frederic Bateman, *op. cit.*, p. 218.
[15] W. Penfield and L. Roberts, *op. cit.*, pp. 60-61.

sensory impressions. This concept of sensory aphasia is as popularly accepted as Broca's motor aphasia.

Twentieth Century Researchers

Marie,[16] 1906, in France, stimulated much controversy in the neurological field by challenging Broca's localization of the speech center. In his opinion, a brain lesion producing loss of speech would not be confined to the motor or expression aspects of speech alone but would affect other areas of language such as reading, writing, spelling, arithmetic and pantomine, as well as general intelligence. He believed that there was only a sensory aphasia and that Broca's aphasia was Wernicke's plus anarthria.

Following the teachings of Jackson, Head accepted and extended the latter's concept that language loss is a disorder in *propositionizing* by stating that the impairment of language by brain damage was an impairment of *symbolic formulation and expression.* Head stated:

> These two aspects of language, the formulation of thought and its skillful expression, although they may be separable as the result of organic lesion of the brain ... in aphasia, both sides are affected, although one may suffer more severely than the other, and I have therefore spoken of these defects in the use of language as disorders of symbolic formulation and expression.[17]

He took strong issue with the extremely mechanical views of localization of Henschen and Kleist. Henschen, discarding all psychological factors, based his study entirely on autopsy material. He started with anatomical facts and deduced from them the specific functional disorders for which they were responsible. Analyzing about 1500 cases, 60 of which he did himself and the rest from literature, he concluded that it was possible to determine a strict localization of speech and related functions. Kleist differentiated various sensory and motor losses as the result of very finely delimited lesions.

[16] Weisenberg and McBride, *Aphasia*, pp. 20-24.
[17] H. Head, *op. cit.*, p. 498.

To Wilson[18] aphasia was a symptom and not a disease. Different types of aphasia could not be referred to as different varieties of disease, but as certain processes of symptoms, all of which were disturbances of speech. While he criticized the "diagram makers", he also took to task the psychologist for neglecting the anatomical and physiological basis of speech.

Von Monakow,[19] 1914, presented his theory of diaschisis to explain the severity of local symptoms following a non-progressive brain lesion and the gradual disappearance of the symptoms after some weeks or months. Essentially, diaschisis consists of a lowering or abolition of the powers of groups of neurones to respond to stimuli within a definite zone of excitation. This zone does not correspond to the usual physiological paths of innervation. It involves only those parts where the fibres from the site of the lesion terminate in primarily uninjured grey matter of the whole central nervous system.

Nielsen approached the problem from the standpoint of cerebral localization not with "the idea of ignoring psychology but while taking it into full account, to stress anatomy and physiology."[20] While accepting Wilson's tri-fold anatomical, physiological and psychological approach as the most worthy of all investigation of aphasia, he used Henschen's data for anatomical support for his position and accepted certain centers as areas of specific function.

Weisenberg and McBride, while accepting the concept of localization to the extent of believing that a lesion in the dominant hemisphere was necessary to produce aphasia, differed from the localizationist "in that we believe that it is impossible to delineate areas for the language function or any of its processes."[21] They found that "aphasia is predominantly a language disorder but that in practically all cases there are alterations in the so-called non-language activities in the reaction to practical situations of daily life and in social responses and attitudes."[22]

[18] S. A. K. Wilson, *Aphasia*, p. 3.
[19] H. Head, *op. cit.*, p. 86.
[20] J. M. Nielson, *op. cit.*, p. 9.
[21] Weisenberg and McBride, *op. cit.*, p. 467.
[22] *Ibid.*, p. 468.

Lashley's findings led him to suggest that "The whole implication of the data is that the higher level integrations are not dependent upon localized structural differentiation but the functions of some more general dynamic organization of the entire cerebral system."[23]

He stressed the idea, however, that in interpreting cortical activity, facts concerning localization as well as mass action should be considered. While he agreed that the occipital region controlled visual functioning and that its destruction would cause a permanent loss of visual functioning, he stated that the capacity to form motor habits is reduced by brain damage in proportion to the extent of destruction and independent of the site of the lesion. *Equipotentiality* is the term he used to describe the ability of the uninjured part of the brain to take over the function of the destroyed part. This phenomenon is subject to the principle of *mass action*. By mass action, Lashley meant that impairment in learning correlated with the extent of mass of extirpated cortex, while the locus of the lesion was inconsequential. This relationship appeared more clearly as the difficulty of the task increased. Likewise, retention of the already acquired habit, was a function of size, not solely of the locus of the cortical lesion.

Franz, an experimental psychologist, reported many studies centered around cortical functioning. While much of his work was done with animals, he also studied the functioning of the human cortex. In this regard, he wrote extensively on the reeducation of the aphasic.[24] Like Goldstein, he did not approve of the use of nonsense syllables as exercises in the reeducation of the aphasic. He started with combinations of sounds that made up simple words, which he believed were more meaningful to the patient and therefore tended to motivate the patient to learn. Franz[25] stressed the importance of strong motivation and emotional incentives on the part of the patient to overcome the physical handicap and bring into action old nerve connections. He concluded from his observa-

[23] K. S. Lashley, "Factors Limiting Recovery after Central Nervous Lesions", p. 741.

[24] S. L. Franz, "Studies in Reeducation: The Aphasias", pp. 349-429.

[25] S. L. Franz, *Nervous and Mental Reeducation.*

tions that the progress made by his patients was due to either the reactivation of old brain connections or the establishment of new ones. In the reeducation of the aphasic, he urged that the instructor take into account the associative losses and try to reestablish these associations. He also recommended that while the therapist should start with the most concrete nouns and proceed to the less concrete, the words that were of the most use to the patient would tend to stimulate the greatest interest and motivation to learn.

A significant contribution to the study of aphasia since about the time of World War I has been the work of Goldstein. He espoused the Gestalt point of view as opposed to that of the localizationists. For him, alterations in personality leading to concrete behavior were evidence of a single basic change in the total personality of patients with cerebral damage.[26] He suggested a relationship between language and thought and pointed out that persons with frontal lobe lesions and those with left cerebral lesions were more likely to show an impairment of the abstract attitude than a person with a right cerebral lesion.[27]

He did not deny that the locus of the lesion determines some manifestations of this basic disturbance, but he believed that basic disturbance followed lesions anywhere in the cerebrum. An adequate examination, he asserted, should cover as many aspects of behavior as possible. In his examinations, he attempted to identify the defects in the ability to reason abstractly. He could not accept localization of performance such as reading, writing, calculation, and speaking. "Every individual speech performance is understandable only from the aspect of its relation to the function of the total organism in its endeavor to realize itself as much as possible in a given situation."[28]

Adhering to the Gestalt approach and principles, regarding the brain functioning of patients with cerebral lesions, Bender stated:

It seems that the gestalt function is more involved the nearer the lesion

[26] K. Goldstein, *The Organism*, p. 1.
[27] K. Goldstein, *After Effects of Brain Injuries in War*, p. 89.
[28] K. Goldstein, *Language and Language Disturbances*, p. 21.

comes to the occipital region. ... Thus, in a general way, we may conclude that the area most probably involved in disturbances of the visual motor gestalt function, as exemplified by these copied test forms, is that between the temporal, parietal and occipital lobes of the dominant hemisphere.[29]

Pascal and Suttell agreed with Bender and pointed out that they observed very little disturbance in the ability to do the Bender designs in subjects with frontal lobotomy or lobectomy. They have observed that:

Circumscribed lesions, especially in the non-dominant hemisphere,result in less disturbance in the ability to reproduce the design than pervasive lesions and acute, confusional states following trauma to the cortex.[30]

Schiller agreed with Goldstein, Head and Jackson that "an aphasic is essentially an individual struggling to readapt himself to the havoc wrought in those parts of the dominant hemisphere which surround the Sylvian Fissure."[31] In his study of 42 patients, he concluded that more than one aspect of speech was affected in each case and that nominal aphasia was present in almost all cases, wherever the wound. He did not believe that the various aspects of language dysfunction could be described in precise terminology.

Blatt[32] found no consistent relationship between the location of a brain lesion and the degree of aphasia. Sudden traumas to the brain, he believed, were responsible for the severity of a language dysfunction rather than the site or extent of a lesion. He concluded that his findings would tend to argue for vicarious functioning of the cerebral cortex and that there was much support for his position in the field of gestalt psychology.

Schuell,[33] during the retraining of aphasics, found an impairment in auditory reception in all his aphasic patients. In his opinion, many of the aphasics' difficulties stemmed from this basic problem

[29] L. Bender, *A Visual Motor Gestalt Test and its Clinical Uses*, p. 75.
[30] G. R. Pascal and B. J. Suttell, *The Bender Gestalt Test*, p. 57.
[31] F. Schiller, "Aphasia Studied in Patients with Missile Wounds", pp. 183-197.
[32] B. Blatt, *The Problem of Language Localization into Specific Brain Areas*, p. 83.
[33] H. Schuell, "Auditory Impairment in Aphasia: Significance and Retraining Techniques", pp. 14-21.

in auditory reception. In a later study, Schuell[34] found that impairment of auditory retention and recall was reversible to a considerable degree; that improvement often resulted from the use of a single therapeutic principle, namely, strong, controlled, intensive auditory stimulation.

Liddell and Phillips rejected the concept of localization and noted that several studies had indicated that "... motor localization investigated by using artificial stimuli bore no fixed relationship to the minor cerebral landmarks which themselves varied unsystematically from species to species and from individual to individual."[35] They pointed out that technical methods and general anaesthesias employed by early researchers were not very adequate and that they still were not perfected. Studies have shown that the same cortical areas yield different motor results depending on the parameter of stimulation and the level of narcosis employed.

In 1936 Penfield found "... evidence of a level of integration within the central nervous system that is higher than that to be found in the cerebral cortex."[36] He located this in the diencephelon and later (1946) included the mesencephelon.

Each functional subdivision of the cerebral cortex of man, according to Penfield and Roberts, may be looked upon as an outgrowth or projection outward of some area of grey matter in the older brain stem. Viewing the organization of the brain in this manner, they thought, was a surer way of predicting functional subdivisions than the cytoarchetectonic approach of Brodman.

Based upon their investigations which involved the use of electrical stimulations to plot brain areas during cerebral surgery, Penfield and Roberts rejected the idea of a localized area for articulate language in Broca's convolution.

We believe that probably the entire third frontal convolution can be excised in the adult with only transient aphasia, provided the remainder

[34] H. Schuell, V. Carroll, B. S. Street, "Clinical Treatment of Aphasia", pp. 43-53.
[35] E. G. T. Liddell and C. G. Phillips, "Thresholds of Cortical Representation", p. 128.
[36] W. Penfield, as reported in W. Penfield and L. Roberts, *op. cit.*, pp. 20-21.

of the hemisphere is functioning normally. So far as our excisions demonstrate, any limited, previously damaged area of the dominant left hemisphere may be excised without producing either immediate or permanent aphasia — providing the remaining brain functions normally.[37]

They concluded:

... the most important area for speech is the posterior temporo-parietal region including the posterior parts of the first, second, and third temporal convolutions behind the vein of Labbe, the supramarginal gyrus, and the angular gyrus. The next important area for speech is that of Broca, including the three gyri anterior to the precentral face area. ... If one of the speech areas is destroyed, then the adjacent areas of cortex and other speech areas function during speech.[38]

However, they believed that the right hemisphere could function for the comprehension of speech only after training.

THE RELATIONSHIP OF BRAIN DAMAGE TO INTELLIGENCE

As has been indicated, Marie thought that true aphasia invariably resulted in a general intellectual deficit as well as in a special defect in language.

Goldstein believed that any damage to the brain affected the volitional attitude more than it did the automatic. When there was an impairment of this volitional attitude, it manifested itself as a personality change which Goldstein called "... impairment of the attitude toward the abstract."[39] A relationship between language, thought and intelligence was suggested in this statement that:

This 'personality' change is to be found especially in cases of lesion of the frontal lobes, but it may also be observed to some extent in cases of lesion of other parts of the cortex. Patients with lesions of the left hemisphere (if they are right-handed people) present this change to a greater degree than patients with right sided lesions.[40]

Eisenson agreed that there was some evidence in support of Goldstein's view that persons with brain damage especially those with

[37] *Ibid.*, pp. 185-186.
[38] *Ibid.*, p. 188.
[39] K. Goldstein, *After Effects of Brain Injuries in War*, p. 88.
[40] *Loc. cit.*

frontal lobe lesions and more often those with left than right cerebral lesion show an impairment of the attitude toward the abstract. However, his own observations made Eisenson question Goldstein's generalization about the loss of abstract attitude in brain-damaged adults. Eisenson believed that such loss was "... generally not as severe as Goldstein has found and that it tends to occur in patients who are past middle age more often than in younger patients."[41] He thought that there was a greater loss of the ability verbally to express the abstract attitude itself and that the adult aphasic was suffering from a relative disinclination to assume and use the abstract attitude, rather than that there was a loss of the abstract attitude itself. Where there was such a loss of abstract functioning, Eisenson found that it was an aggravation of a premorbid tendency rather than a new feature of the patient's behavior. He disagreed with Goldstein's concept that concretism was a permanent change of personality which was found especially in cases with frontal lobe lesions. Usually this was found in persons past middle age who had old lesions. Where concretism did occur, Eisenson believed it was an attitude that the patient assumed and made habitual unless it was changed through early training or strong motivation.

Eisenson considered aphasia *defective symbol behavior* that manifested itself by defects in internal symbol processes (thinking) as well as in external symbol processes (speaking, reading, writing). The symbols that present the difficulty may be linguistic or non-linguistic. Like Goldstein he believed the total organism must be considered in aphasia because there were, besides the language disturbance, modifications in thinking, attitude and personality, as well as overt behavioral changes in the intellectual and emotional spheres. However, many disturbances of the aphasic "are part of the over-all picture of 'organicity' which the aphasic as well as the non-aphasic brain-damaged person manifests. Included in this picture are disturbances in attention, memory, perseveration, rigidity and orderliness; also concretism, catastrophic response, euphoria and withdrawal tendencies."[42]

[41] Jon Eisenson, *Examining for Aphasia*, p. 3.
[42] *Ibid.*, pp. 7-11.

In a study of right-handed non-aphasics who suffered damage of the right cerebral hemisphere, employing a variety of language tests, Eisenson[43] found that there was a modification of language and intellectual ability, especially on tasks involving abstract concepts.

Appelbaum[44] compared a group of brain-damaged non-aphasic adults with a *psychiatric* and a *normal* group on a 60-word Word Association test. He found that the brain-damaged group showed significantly more repetitions, blocking, etc., than the other two groups and that organics could be separated from non-organics by the test.

In both of these last two studies there is an impairment of language ability even though the lesion is in the non-dominant right cerebral hemisphere and the patients are classified as *non-aphasic.*

Wepman's[45] findings supported Eisenson's position that it was not usual for brain-injured patients to demonstrate an absolute loss of the capacity to abstract or that this loss, when demonstrated, was permanent. He found that the brain deficit which produced the aphasia was responsible for many far-reaching symptoms beyond the realm of language. For him, many personality aberrations, many atypical modes of behavior and various other symptoms of a functional nature were direct or indirect results of the cerebral impairment and were due to a disturbance in the integrating capacity of the cortex. As a result, Wepman developed a holistic approach which led to the treatment of the individual rather than the treatment of the disorder. In a subsequent article, Wepman[46] formulated three concepts involved in the recovery from aphasia. They were stimulation, facilitation and motivation. He believed that therapy that was supportive as well as instructive was the only way in which aphasics could regain a wholesome self-concept and that the content of the therapy was less important than the manner in which it

[43] Jon Eisenson, "Language and Intellectual Modifications Associated with Right Cerebral Damage", pp. 49-53.

[44] S. A. Appelbaum, "Expanded Word Test as a Measure of Psychological Deficit Associated with Brain Damage", pp. 78-84.

[45] J. M. Wepman, *Recovery from Aphasia*, pp. 24, 70-75.

[46] J. M. Wepman, "A Conceptual Model for the Processes Involved in Recovery from Aphasia", pp. 4-13.

was conducted. He found that while there was a measurable loss of I.Q. after injury, this loss was frequently not permanent and could be reversed through training.

Hebb pointed out that "... aphasia is by no means a mere loss of speech; the patient has lost something else as well, an intellectual capacity. ..."[47]

There have been studies that have questioned the concept that there is a relationship between language and intellectual functioning.

Kennedy and Wolf[48] believed that a distinction should be made between aphasia and intellectual factors.

A study done by Meyers[49] supported this position by finding that dysphasic patients did no worse in certain non-language problem-solving situations than did control patients.

Reitan found no difference on the Rorschach[50] test between dysphasic and non-dysphasic patients. On the Wechsler Mental Abilities Scale[51] and the Wechsler Bellevue Scale Form 1,[52] the dysphasic did better on the performance tests but the differences were not statistically significant and the non-dysphasic did significantly better on the verbal tests except for Arithmetic where the difference was not statistically significant.

Bauer and Becka concluded that aphasic patients did not demonstrate greater impairment of abstract ability than did other brain-lesion patients. They found that right lesion patients scored lower on non-language intellectual tasks than left lesion patients. They could neither confirm nor contradict the concept that patients with frontal lesions showed greater impairment than patients with non-

[47] D. O. Hebb, *The Organization of Behavior*, p. 161.

[48] F. Kennedy and A. Wolf, "The Relationship of Intellect to Speech Defect in Aphasic Patients", pp. 125-145.

[49] R. Meyers, "Relation of Thinking and Language; an Experimental Approach Using Dysphasic Patients", p. 112.

[50] Ralph M. Reitan, "Intellectual Functions in Aphasic and Non-Aphasic Brain-Injured Subjects", pp. 202-212.

[51] Ralph M. Reitan, "Intelligence and Language Functions in Dysphasic Patients", pp. 2-8.

[52] Ralph M. Reitan, "Certain Differential Effects of Left and Right Cerebral Lesions in Human Adults", pp. 474-478.

frontal lesions. Their results indicated that Goldstein's conclusion that left hemisphere lesion cases were more damaged with respect to abstract functions was not confirmed, "... the converse was shown to be more credible."[53] Bauer and Becka found also that the lesion locus might make for a differential impairment in the tactual, visual and auditory modality.

Williams *et. al.*,[54] tested 64 brain-damaged patients in the age range of eighteen to fifty years. They concluded that traumatic brain damage resulted in a general deficit in intelligence test scores with little differential deficit. They found that reading, vocabulary, arithmetical reasoning, and clerical speed scores declined slightly more than spatial tests, pattern analysis, and mechanical aptitude.

While Blatt's findings indicated a lowering of intellectual functioning in aphasia as measured by a standardized performance technique, he could not determine how much of this to attribute to the amount of tissue destroyed and how much to the location of the lesion in the dominant hemisphere. However the evidence seemed to "... argue for a relationship between amount of functional cortical tissue and intellectual functioning when the tissue destruction is extensive."[55]

Aita *et. al.*,[56] after concluding that the Wechsler Mental Ability Scale was the most efficient diagnostic tool of the tests studied, reported that scores on Arithmetic, Comprehension, Picture Arrangement, Digit Symbol and Block Design were lowered by brain injury. They found that brain-injured cases are characterized by visuo-motor disturbances, loss of ability to shift, possible memory defects, loss in capacities involving abstraction, organization, synthesis, analysis, and also showed reduced learning capacity. There was also an increase in rigidity, perseveration and stereotyped thought. Their results confirmed the findings of Goldstein, Scheerer,

[53] R. W. Bauer and D. M. Becka, "Intellect after Cerebro-vascular Accident", p. 380.

[54] A. L. Williams, A. Lubin, C. F. Geisking, "Direct Measurement of Cognitive Deficit".

[55] B. Blatt, *op. cit.*, p. 84.

[56] J. A. Aita, S. G. Armitage, R. M. Reitan, and A. Rabinowitz, "The Use of Certain Psychological Tests in Evaluation of Brain Injury", pp. 25-44.

and others, that brain-injured patients tend to function on a lower level, and that the personality is organized as a new gestalt enabling it to cope more adequately with the trauma, even though on a lower, more concrete, more rigid and circumscribed level.

That the lowered functioning of the brain-damaged patient may be due to factors other than organic or physiological changes has been demonstrated. Several studies have indicated the impact and significance of psychological factors such as anxiety and other emotional overlays on the performance of aphasics. Kennedy[57] reported the case of a veteran in treatment who showed marked improvement in speech. The main emphasis of the therapy was on maintaining a good rapport between the therapist and the patient. The therapist found that the severe anxiety resulting from a sense of frustration brought on by the aphasic impediment, retarded the process of relearning. In another study, it was found that even when there were segments of the brain preserved, with the capacity for relearning, the emotional overlay resulting from the brain trauma prevented or retarded language recovery.[58] Linn and Stern state: "The impairment of function in organic brain disease is the resultant of two factors; the actual structural damage incurred and the emotional responses to the illness."[59] They found that the emotional responses to the illness resulted in a reduced functioning and withdrawal of the aphasic. The administering of sodium amytal brought about an immediate improvement in all patients. The drug, it was explained, removed the inhibitory effects of anxiety which tended to reduce functioning. The patients were encouraged by their initial success in expressing themselves and seemed capable of more effort as well as being better motivated toward the possibility of rehabilitation. On the other hand, Bergman and Green found that "Administration of sodium amytal did not improve the speech of any patient in this series over periods of observation,

[57] L. Kennedy, "Remedial Procedures for Handling Aphasic Patients", pp. 646-699.

[58] N. Blackman and L. L. Tureen, "Aphasia; a Psychosomatic Approach in Rehabilitation", pp. 193-196.

[59] L. Linn and M. Stern, "Sodium Amytal in Treatment of Aphasia", p. 705.

ranging from a few weeks to several months."[60] Billows concluded that since the improvement seemed temporary, it would be difficult at this stage to come to any conclusions as to the efficacy of the drug and that further studies were required.[61]

There have been several studies that indicate that positive results can be achieved by treating emotional factors in aphasia by psychotherapy. Chenven reported that:

Plateaus in the recovery process due to either age, etiology, or onset of illness do not seem to be supported when group therapy is provided along with language retraining. Older patients, ill many years due to cerebrovascular accidents, all of which have been considered negative aspects for adequate recovery, made considerable progress.[62]

Blackman, working with veterans, concluded that group psychotherapy was an important adjunct in the treatment and supervision of head injury cases. He stated:

The head injury patient will continue to adjust and improve for a long time, especially if a favorable understanding of his problems were available, a keen interest in his progress was maintained and a warm, sympathetic and encouraging attitude was evinced.[63]

Aronson, *et. al.* (1956), employing group therapy with a heterogeneous group of aphasic veterans reported that:

... the group responded quite favorably toward the program as a whole and towards the manner in which it was conducted and expressed a need to continue with it.[64]

THE RELATIONSHIP OF LANGUAGE TO THOUGHT

Bastian began his first paper in 1869 with the statement that one thinks in words. "In amnesia, there is an inability to recall words,

[60] P. Bergman and M. Green, "Aphasia; Effect of Intravenous Sodium Amytal", p. 475.

[61] B. W. Billows, "Observation of the Use of Sodium Amytal in the Treatment of Aphasia", p. 12.

[62] H. Chenven, *Effects of Group Therapy Upon Language Recovery in Predominantly Expressive Aphasia*, pp. 156-157.

[63] N. Blackman, "Group Psychotherapy with Aphasics", p. 160.

[64] M. Aronson, L. Shotin, and J. C. Cook, "Socio-Psycho-Therapeutic Approach to the Treatment of Aphasic Patients", pp. 358-359.

i.e., they cannot properly be revived in the auditory perceptive centers, and there is an almost proportional impairment of the thinking powers."[65]

As early as 1866, Jackson indicated that a person does not speak or think in words or signs only, but in words or signs referring to one another in a particular manner. While Jackson agreed that words serve not only in speech but in thought, he rejected the concept that thought was internal speech. Speech, he believed, was only a part of thought which may or may not be exteriorized, but the man who was speechless could think. He summed up by stating:

In short there is intact in the speechless man all the processes he ever had for the recognition of objects which is putting ideas of objects, if I may so speak, in propositional order. The speechless man has lost speech only.[66]

He continued:

Although he has but one side for verbalizing, the automatic side, he has according to my hypothesis, two sides for the revival of images, thus he can still think, can have certain relations of likeness and unlikeness. No doubt he is lame in his thinking. He will be unable to keep before himself the results of complex arrangements of images. He can bring two images into coexistence, in one unit of time, but cannot without speech, organize the connexion if it be one of difficulty.[67]

Combining the disorders of language produced by a unilateral lesion of the brain under the general heading of *symbolic formulation and expression*, Head pointed out that "Thus the patient may have profound difficulty in manipulating visual images at will for the purposes of verbal expression, although he can employ them with ease in other modes of thinking. It is not images as such that are disturbed, but images used in a certain manner directed towards a definite end."[68] He believed that it was not the *general intellectual capacity* which was primarily affected, but the mechanisms by which certain aspects of mental activity were brought into play.

[65] H. Head, *op. cit.*, p. 115.
[66] *Ibid.*, p. 96.
[67] *Ibid.*, pp. 98-99.
[68] *Ibid.*, p. 210.

However, in so far as these processes were necessary for the perfect exercise of mental aptitudes, general intelligence undoubtedly suffered.

Head concluded that while some types of thinking were dependent on language formulation, others were independent of it.

> Thought presupposes the existence of language but exceeds it widely in range and there are many forms of behavior, the results of thinking, which do not require the intervention of a symbol. Percepts and emotions alone may determine the form of the response.[69]

Watson, the founder of Behaviorism, believed that language and thought were inseparable.

> The behaviorist advances the view that *what the psychologists have hitherto called thought is in short nothing but talking to ourselves.*[70]

He thought that the verbal process whenever it was present always was an actual functioning part of every act of skill. The unitary concept of behavior and thought is clearly expressed in the following:

> I have several times maintained that when an individual reacts to an object or situation, his whole body reacts. For us, this means that manual organization, language organization, (after it begins) and visceral organization all function together — each and every time the body reacts.[71]

LATERALIZATION OF CEREBRAL FUNCTION

In 1865, Broca summarized a case of a 47 year old left-handed female who had had epilepsy and right hemiparesis since infancy. Although she had never suffered any speech disturbance, at autopsy, a large lesion in the distribution of the left middle cerebral artery was revealed. Broca assumed that the right hemisphere had taken over the speech function and then generalized that the right hemisphere is dominant for speech in all left-handed people.

[69] Henry Head, *op. cit.*, p. 519.
[70] J. B. Watson, *Behaviorism*, p. 199.
[71] *Ibid.*, p. 202.

Thus was created the dogma that the right cerebral hemisphere is dominant for speech in the left handed, in the same way that the left cerebral hemisphere is dominant for the right handed individual.

While Jackson (1868) was the first to report a case of a left-handed man with a lesion of the right hemisphere and aphasia, he seemed to have accepted Broca's theory on it. However, as has been indicated previously, he believed that both hemispheres of the brain functioned in the production of speech and thought. He did not think they duplicated each other. He stated:

> 1) that both halves are alike insofar as each contains processes for words; 2) that they are unlike in that the left is for the use of words only in speech, and the right for other processes in which words serve.[72]

In short, Jackson thought that the left half of the brain is that by which we speak, the right is the half by which we receive propositions.

Lashley[73] conceptualized a dynamic organization of the entire cerebral system and used the term *equipotentiality* to describe the ability of the uninjured part of the brain to take over the function of the destroyed part.

Although Nielsen espoused the theory of the localization of cerebral function, in a more recent report on a training program with aphasic veterans, he concluded, "Given fairly good health and one good hemisphere for retraining, virtually any aphasic can obtain satisfactory results in a retraining program."[74]

Esti Freud accepted the concepts of Jackson, Pick, Head, and Goldstein. He doubted that the brain had the capacity of restitution of damaged or lost tissue but believed that "... in the neighboring lobes of the brain, cerebral tissue may be present vastly in excess of the actual need and that in addition various localities are available for the same purpose. ..."[75]

[72] H. Head, *op. cit.*, p. 81.
[73] K. S. Lashley, *op. cit.*, p. 79.
[74] J. M. Nielsen, "Aphasia Rehabilitation: A Report of Nine Successful Cases", pp. 461-469.
[75] Esti D. Freud, "Clinical Language Rehabilitation of Veterans, Methods and Results", p. 887.

E. Freud concluded:

The results obtained in the clinics with aphasia patients confirm Pavlov's findings. He demonstrated more or less conclusively that the cortex is a mosaic of function in which nothing is permanently fixed except motor and various sensory areas ... that it is a kaleidoscope with the infiinite possibilities of inhibition, adaptation and substitution in mental and emotional processes.[76]

Bauer and Wepman[77] took issue with Nielsen who believed that the right (minor) hemisphere could assume the function of language after the left (major) hemisphere was damaged. They found that the recovery of language was more likely to result from the development of function in additional areas of the damaged left hemisphere when specialized nerve tissue was available. Only when the destruction of the left hemisphere was complete was there a likelihood of total transfer. Language symbolization, they stated, was a function of the integration of the cortical and subcortical nervous system rather than of the cortex itself. Symbolization recovery depended upon the cortex reassuming the integrative hierarchial control over the subcortex and not upon total migration.

Bauer and Wepman questioned the commonly accepted relationship between handedness, focal lesions in the cortex, and language disturbances after cerebral trauma. They concluded that cerebral dominance appeared to be unique to the left hemisphere. They found the left hemisphere involved in the symbolic language act in practically all the subjects studied. Intellectual functions not involving language appear to be particularly impaired with right hemisphere lesions. These include such functions as social and ideational comprehension, visual-motor planning, patterning and reproduction, auditory patterning and arithmetic computation.

Heilbrun[78] found that left cerebral lesion patients demonstrated greater impairment on verbal tests as compared to right lesion patients. However, he could not support his hypothesis that

[76] *Ibid.*, p. 889.

[77] R. W. Bauer and J. M. Wepman, "Lateralization of Cerebral Functions", p. 176.

[78] A. B. Heilbrun, Jr., "Psychological Test Performance as a Function of Lateral Localization of Cerebral Lesion", pp. 10-11.

right lesion patients would demonstrate greater impairment on spatial batteries. He did find that the two intra-group battery patterns were significantly different.

However, Levitt, *et. al.*, in a study of 41 male Veterans Administration patients reported "... the right sided group was found to be consistently inferior to the left-sided group on each of the non-verbal task variables."[79]

To determine the differences in response to structured, usual stimuli, Wood[80] compared a group of right hemiplegics with a group of left hemiplegics (ages 10 to 30 years old). She found no positive relationship between the side of the brain in which the lesion occurred and a disturbance in visual perception.

In a study where only lateralization of function was investigated, Reitan employed the Wechsler-Bellevue Scale (Form 1) on subjects that were divided into three groups. His results revealed that:

> On each of the verbal subtests the group with lesions of the left hemisphere had the lowest means. On the performance subtests, however, the group with lesions of the right hemisphere consistently had the lowest mean scores. The group with diffuse brain damage roughly approximated the group with lesions of the right hemisphere on the verbal subtests and the group with lesions of the left hemisphere on the performance subtests.[81]

Anderson did a statistical analysis of the Wechsler-Bellevue Intelligence Test subtest differences between the performances of brain-damaged patients with dominant hemisphere lesions and non-dominant hemisphere lesions. He observed that dominant hemisphere brain-damaged patients demonstrated greater losses on verbal abilities, while non-dominant hemisphere brain-damaged patients showed greater losses on performance tasks. He concluded that the dominant hemisphere brain-damaged patient *forgets what to do* while the non-dominant hemisphere brain-

[79] Herbert Levitt, *et. al.* "The Laterality Hypothesis in the Assessment of Localized Brain Damage", p. 180.

[80] Nancy E. Wood, "A Comparison of Right Hemiplegics with Left Hemiplegics in Visual Perception", pp. 370-380.

[81] Ralph M. Reitan, "Certain Differential Effects of Left and Right Cerebral Lesions in Human Adults", p. 475.

damaged patient *forgets how to do*.[82] Since eight of the fourteen patients in the group with lesions of the left hemisphere had a mild residual dysphasia, there was a possibility that the impaired performance on the verbal subtests was associated with organic language loss. However, Anderson found it difficult to say whether the verbal scores represented an impairment in intelligence or to use Goldstein's term, a defect in the instrumentalities of speech.

In an investigation of laterality of cerebral function, Stark employed three groups of twenty subjects each. One group had lesions of the left cerebral hemisphere, the second had lesions of the right cerebral hemisphere and the third was a normal control group without any known cerebral damage. Using paired-associate learning tasks, she found that the right hemisphere lesion group did as well as the control group on the verbal tasks but scored on the average eleven more errors on the visual-spatial tasks. The left hemisphere lesion group did almost as well as the control group on the visual-spatial tasks but scored on the average eleven more errors on the verbal tasks. While none of the mean differences were statistically significant between the experimental and control groups, the mean differences between the experimental groups were significant by *t*-test at greater than the .01 level. Stark concluded that, "At an empirical level, the results of the present study suggest some clear relationship regarding localization of cerebral functioning."[83]

Summary

Historically, many significant writings and researches in the areas of brain organization and functioning started with the turn of the nineteenth century. Since many of these investigations were based upon studies of brain-damaged patients the researches broadened out to include the problems of the relationship between brain-

[82] A. Lloyd Anderson, "The Effect of Laterality Localization of Focal Brain Lesions on the Wechsler-Bellevue Subtests", pp. 149-153.

[83] R. Stark, "An Investigation of Unilateral Cerebral Pathology with Equated Verbal and Visual-Spatial Tasks", p. 285.

damage and intelligence, brain-damage and recovery, language and thought, and the lateralization of cerebral functioning.

Despite the prolific writings and investigations of numerous researchers, no unified or generally accepted theory has emerged. The theories of brain functioning range from the extreme localizationists such as those of Broca, Wernicke, and Nielsen to the *mass action* and *equipotentiality* theories of Lashley and the Gestalt theories of Goldstein. In the areas of the relationship of brain-damage to intelligence, there are various theories, as demonstrated by the positions of such researchers as Marie and Goldstein who believed that there is a close relationship and that brain-damage makes for a general intellectual deficit, while Eisenson and Wepman thought that brain-damage made for a selective type of intellectual impairment. In the area of the relationship of language to thought, similar disagreements existed. Bastian and Watson found a very close relationship between the two but this was denied by Jackson, Head, Kennedy and Wolf. The questions of cerebral dominance, handedness, and the ability of one cerebral hemisphere to take over the function of the other hemisphere, or one part of the brain to take over the function of another part of the brain still have to be resolved. While Broca thought that cerebral dominance was related to handedness, Bauer and Wepman questioned this relationship. They, also, took issue with Nielsen who believed that the right hemisphere could assume the function of language after the left hemisphere was damaged.

The one conclusion that seems to stem from this multiplicity of theories and concepts is that there is still a great need for further research in this vital area of the human organism, namely, the cerebral cortex.

2. PURPOSE OF THE INVESTIGATION

THE PROBLEM

General Statement

The problem of this study is to determine and evaluate the effect of language disturbance on intellectual functioning among brain-damaged individuals.

The research is concerned with a comparison of the performance of hemiplegic patients with aphasia and hemiplegic patients without aphasia in the age range of the fifties and sixties on non-verbal tasks of intellectual functioning. The tasks involve closure, space visualization, spatial orientation, adaptive flexibility, and memory.

Specific Problems

The specific problems of the research are:

1. To determine the extent of language facility and non-verbal intellectual functioning in hemiplegic patients with aphasia. This group is designated the Aphasic group.
2. To determine the extent of language facility and non-verbal intellectual functioning in hemiplegic patients without aphasia. This group is designated the Non-aphasic group.
3. To make intra- and inter-group comparisons of the two research populations on the basis of the data obtained in sub-problems one and two.

Delimitations

The population of this study consists of two groups of adult hemiplegic patients, one group with aphasia, the other group without aphasia. Each group is composed of fifteen patients.

The patients had been diagnosed on admission to the hospital by the admitting physician as *cerebral vascular accidents* resulting in hemiplegia with aphasia or in hemiplegia without aphasia.

All but three of the patients were made available from the in-patient population of the Bird S. Coler Hospital and Home. The remaining three were from the in-patient population of Bellevue Hospital. Both these installations are New York City hospitals under the supervision and control of the New York City Department of Hospitals. All the patients were indigent residents of New York City. The patients were agreeable to and capable of participating in the testing procedure. All had been able to understand English premorbidly.

The patients ranged in age from 52 years to 67 years with a medical record of no more than one cerebro-vascular accident and were able to ambulate or to be transported by wheelchair. They were not on an active rehabilitation program.

BASIC ASSUMPTIONS

It is assumed that individuals differ in levels of intellectual functioning.

It is further assumed that the devices used in this study to evaluate language and non-verbal performance tasks of intellectual functioning are adequate measures of the various specified areas of functioning.

BASIC HYPOTHESIS

Rationale for the Hypothesis

Goldstein, Jackson, and Head, as well as other suggest a relationship between language and abstract functioning. Watson goes even further and makes a complete identification between language and thought. He states that, "... thought is in short nothing but talking to ourselves."[1]

Kennedy and Wolf question the above relationship. They find that,

> There is a distinction between intellectual defect and aphasia, that thought is possible without speech or word, that defective speech can exist as something apart from intelligence, ideation, attention, memory and powers of association.[2]

Subsequent studies with non-language performance tasks done by Meyers and by Bauer and Becka support Kennedy and Wolf's position. In a series of three investigations, Reitan rejects any relationship between language and nonverbal intellectual functioning.

If language is related to intellectual functioning, then the loss of language ability through brain injury should make for a greater impairment of ability to perform intellectual tasks than a brain injury without an impairment of language functioning.

In this study, it is hypothesized that no consistent relationship exists between ability to engage in non-verbal intellectual tasks and language disturbance.

If this view is correct it may be inferred that: The non-aphasic group will demonstrate no significant superiority over the aphasic group on tests and measures of non-verbal performance tasks of intellectual functioning.

[1] J. B. Watson, *Behaviorism*, p. 199.

[2] F. Kennedy and A. Wolf, "The Relationship of Intellect to Speech Defect in Aphasic Patients", p. 143.

3. PROCEDURE IN COLLECTING THE DATA

SETTING

The data for this research were collected at the Bird S. Coler Hospital and Home on Welfare Island and at Bellevue Hospital. Both installations are New York City Hospitals, under the supervision and control of the New York City Department of Hospitals.

Bird S. Coler Hospital and Home is a 2000 bed rehabilitation center. It provides a diversified program for children and adult male and female patients with various types of physical disabilities. There is an active rehabilitation program with a capacity for 200 patients. Sheltered workshops are also available for those patients who are willing and able to participate. The program at this center is intended to assist the patients in recouping as much of their losses as possible and to aid them in achieving a level of functioning as close to their maximum potential as possible.

Upon admission to this center, the patients usually have passed through the acute stage of their illnesses. Approximately 70 per cent of the patients admitted suffer from neurological disabilities. Many patients, after completing the rehabilitation program, remain in the Home and are provided with custodial care. Some patients return to their families, while other patients are placed in nursing homes or other facilities.

For the purpose of achieving an effective, total approach, the professional staff in the rehabilitation program is organized into teams. These teams represent a variety of disciplines; included among them are medical doctors, psychiatrists, nurses, physical therapists, occupational therapists, speech therapists, social service workers, vocational counselors and psychologists.

The Department of Physical Medicine and Rehabilitation at

Bellevue Hospital consists of two wards, one male and the other female. Its services, staff and approach are similar to that outlined above for Bird S. Coler Hospital and Home but on a more limited scale.

POPULATIONS INVOLVED IN THE RESEARCH

Most of the patients for this study were obtained from the in-patient population of the Bird S. Coler Hospital and Home. In addition to the Bird S. Coler population, three patients were drawn from the in-patient rehabilitation service at Bellevue Hospital.

All the patients in the wards at Bird S. Coler Hospital and Home and in the two wards at Bellevue Hospital who met the delimitations of this research were accepted. The selection of the patients was based upon an examination of their medical records, followed by a personal interview by the researcher to determine whether they met the delimitations of this study. The delimitations, as indicated above, are: the patients had been diagnosed on admission to the hospital by the admitting physician as *cerebral vascular accidents* (CVA) resulting in hemiplegia with aphasia or hemiplegia without aphasia; the patients were all on the in-patient service; they ranged in age between 50 years and 70 years; there was no medical record of any previous C.V.A.; they had been able to understand English premorbidly; they were not on an active rehabilitation program; they were able to ambulate or be transported by wheelchair; they were agreeable to and capable of participating in the testing procedure.

Thirty cerebrovascular accident (CVA) patients were employed in this study, divided into two groups. One group consisted of fifteen patients diagnosed on admission into the hospital as cerebrovascular accident with hemiplegia and aphasia, hereafter referred to as the Aphasic Group. The other group consisted of fifteen patients diagnosed on admission to the hospital as cerebrovascular accident with hemiplegia but without aphasia, hereafter referred to as the Non-aphasic group.

Table I presents pertinent identifying data regarding the patients in the aphasic and non-aphasic groups.

All the patients were examined by the researcher in the office during the usual working hours for that installation, which are from 9 A.M. to 5 P.M., from Monday to Friday, inclusive. The subjects were seen for one hour testing sessions for as many times as required for them to complete the battery of tests. Uniform testing conditions were maintained for all the subjects.

Population Variables Equated

There is evidence that intelligence tests results may be influenced by such factors as age, sex, duration of disability, socio-economic and educational background. In this regard, Hebb has pointed out:

> Now test scores are related to education, social background, and occupation, a concatenation that can be summarized as the factor of sophistication. Scores are also affected by age, rising to a peak in the teens and declining (for almost all tests) after the twenties. These are the correlates of intelligence in normal persons, as far as is known at present.[1]

Since these variables may influence the results on tests of intellectual functioning with a brain-damaged population, they were controlled in this study.

Table I shows that the sex distribution for both groups is equivalent.

Owing to the nature of the types of institutions involved in this research, both city hospitals, the socio-economic background of the subjects were for the most part similar. All the patients in this study were indigent New York City residents coming from the lower socio-economic class. This is indicated also by the vocational background of the patients as shown in Table I.

To determine whether any statistically significant differences existed between the two groups in relation to the variables of age, education and duration of disability, these variables were submitted to the *t*-test.

1 D. O. Hebb, *The Organization of Behavior*, p. 279.

Group Identification, Sex, Age, Education, I
of Birth and Years Lived in the U.S.A. of t

Subject Number	Group Identification[a]	Sex	Age	Education Years
1	A	M	55	12
2	A	F	67	6
3	A	F	66	4
4	A	M	65	0
5	A	M	62	7
6	A	M	55	6
7	A	M	56	10
8	A	F	53	8
9	A	F	65	8
10	A	M	58	8
11	A	M	65	8
12	A	M	64	8
13	A	F	54	12
14	A	M	60	12
15	A	M	63	6
16	NA	F	57	2
17	NA	M	58	8
18	NA	F	58	8
19	NA	M	55	6
20	NA	M	56	8
21	NA	M	61	8
22	NA	M	65	12
23	NA	M	67	8
24	NA	F	62	8
25	NA	M	52	8
26	NA	F	61	8
27	NA	M	61	0
28	NA	M	63	6
29	NA	F	67	9
30	NA	M	60	5

[a] A = Aphasic
NA = Non-Aphasic

)isability, Vocational Background, Country
4phasic and Fifteen Non-Aphasic Patients

·ation of ty in Months	Vocational Background	Country of Birth	Years in U.S.A.
180	Masseur	U.S.A.	55
19	Housewife	U.S.A.	67
140	Domestic	B.W.I.	60
3	Waiter	Turkey	52
24	Porter	B.W.I.	57
48	Bartender	Ireland	32
18	Elec. Worker	U.S.A.	55
20	Needlepoint Worker	U.S.A.	53
28	Store Clerk	U.S.A.	65
60	Toolmaker	U.S.A.	58
12	Toolmaker	U.S.A.	65
132	Metal Worker	B.W.I.	45
108	Housewife	U.S.A.	54
65	Cabinet Maker	U.S.A.	60
36	Chauffeur	U.S.A.	63
27	Factory Floorwalker	B.W.I.	44
12	Clerical Worker	U.S.A.	58
48	Cleaning Woman	U.S.A.	58
6	Building Sup't.	U.S.A.	55
36	Brokerage Clerk	U.S.A.	56
97	Machinist	U.S.A.	61
228	Railroad Worker	U.S.A.	65
31	Restaurant Bar Boy	U.S.A.	67
19	Factory Floorwalker	U.S.A.	62
14	Factory Handyman	Germany	30
66	Housewife	U.S.A.	61
60	Unskilled Worker	Poland	42
132	Chauffeur	U.S.A.	63
54	Housewife	U.S.A.	67
24	Cabinet Maker	Italy	48

The following formula, for small independent samples was used for testing the null hypothesis.[2]

$$t = \frac{\bar{X}_1 - \bar{X}_2}{S\bar{x}_1 - \bar{x}_2}$$

$$\text{where } S\bar{x}_1 - \bar{x}_2 = \sqrt{\left(\frac{\Sigma x_1^2 + \Sigma x_2^2}{N_1 + N_2 - 2}\right)\left(\frac{1}{N_1} + \frac{1}{N_2}\right)}$$

$$\text{and where } \Sigma x_1^2 = \Sigma X_1^2 - \frac{(\Sigma X_1)^2}{N_1}$$

To determine whether one group was more variable than the other on the variables of age, education, and duration of disability, the F-test was applied using the formula $F = \frac{S_1^2}{S_2^2}$

The F-ratio was established by dividing the smaller variance into the larger.[3] The results of these tests are indicated in Table II.

Age. — Wechsler has pointed out that "The decline of mental ability with age is part of the general senescent process of the organism as a whole."[4] Pascal and Suttell concluded that, while between the ages of fifteen and fifty, age had little effect on Bender Gestalt scores, "Qualitatively, we feel certain of a definite relationship between age and B-G score for the older age groups although we do not have sufficient data to prove our point."[5] Stark found such a significant positive correlation of age with visual-spatial scores, that she concluded: "Hence, visual-spatial tests of cerebral pathology should be carefully equated for age if they are to have any validity."[6]

The subjects in this study ranged in age from fifty-two to sixty-seven, as is shown in Table I.

The results of the t-test and F-test are shown in Table II. A t of .16 is not statistically significant at the .05 level, and the null

[2] Allen L. Edwards, *Statistical Methods for the Behavioral Sciences*, p. 253.
[3] *Ibid.*, pp. 271-273.
[4] D. Wechsler, *The Measurement of Adult Intelligence*, p. 57.
[5] G. R. Pascal and B. Suttell, *The Bender Gestalt Test*, p. 22.
[6] R. Stark, "An Investigation of Unilateral Cerebral Pathology with Equated Verbal and Visual-Spatial Tasks", p. 286.

hypothesis is supported. The two groups do not differ significantly in relation to age. An *F* of 1.34 is not statistically significant at the .05 level, indicating no statistically significant difference in variability in the variable of age for the groups.

TABLE II

Mean, Standard Deviation, F-test Scores and t-test Scores for the Variables of Age, Education and Duration of Disability of the Fifteen Aphasic and Fifteen Non-Aphasic Patients

Variable	Group[a]	Mean	Standard Deviation	*F*-test[b]	*t*-test[c]
Age	A	60.47	5.00	1.34	.16 (N.S.)
	NA	60.20	4.31		
Education	A	7.67	3.20	1.23	.66 (N.S.)
	NA	6.93	2.89		
Duration of Disability	A	4.95	4.60	1.11	.09 (N.S.)
	NA	4.79	4.85		

[a] A = Aphasic; NA = Non-Aphasic
[b] For each F; d.f. = 14 and 14; F.05 = 2.48; F.01 = 3.70
[c] d.f. = 28; t.05 = 2.048; t.01 = 2.763 (N.S.) = Not significant

Education. — Again, as in the variable of age, the education variable is highly correlated to intelligence. Wechsler stated:

Practically all studies show that educational attainment (as measured by the number of years of school attendance) and intelligence ratings (as measured by test scores) correlate to a relatively high degree. The correlation ranges in most cases from .60 to .80.[7]

The education of the subjects in this study ranged from zero years to twelve years. Table I lists the education in number of years successfully completed for each subject. As indicated in Table II, a t of .66 is not statistically significant at the .05 level and the null hypothesis that the two groups are not different in relation to education is supported. An F of 1.23 is not statistically significant at the .05 level retaining the null hypothesis concerning variance.

Duration of Disability. — This variable is most significant during the early stages of illness following a cerebrovascular accident. For the first six months post trauma, improvements in functioning usually occur in the patient. This has been referred to as *spontaneous recovery.*[8] Table I indicates the number of months from the onset of illness to the time of testing for each patient. Table II shows a t of .09 which is not significant at the .05 level and the null hypothesis is retained for this factor. As for the variance, an F of 1.11 is not significant at the .05 level and the null hypothesis is retained.

The results of this statistical analysis demonstrate that the two groups are equated for the factors of age, sex, duration of disability, socio-economic and educational background.

Wechsler has pointed out that:

> Although the correlation between educational attainment and intelligence level is high, it does not necessarily follow that the latter is dependent upon the former. It might also mean that the education which an individual is capable of attaining is dependent upon his intelligence.[9]

In view of the lack of any statistically significant differences in education, as well as all the other variables for the groups, the inference may be drawn that there was no statistically significant difference between the groups premorbidly in the ability to function intellectually.

[7] D. Wechsler, *op. cit.*, p. 103.
[8] E. Butfield and O. Zangwill, "Re-education in Aphasia", pp. 75-79.
[9] D. Wechsler, *op. cit.*, pp. 103-104.

TESTS AND OTHER EVALUATIVE DEVICES

A battery of one language test and four non-verbal performance tests was administered to each subject. In addition, a memory score and an adaptive flexibility score were determined.

Eisenson Test for Aphasia[10]

The Eisenson Test was employed to evaluate the level of language facility in each subject. This instrument is frequently used in clinics for the measurement of language ability in aphasia and has been employed in researches for this purpose. Chenven[11] employed the Eisenson Test to evaluate the language ability and defects in his research population. His study was concerned with the effect of group psychotherapy as an adjunct to speech therapy with a group of expressive aphasic patients. Blatt[12] used the Eisenson Test in his investigation concerned with language localization into specific brain areas. Studying a group of brain-damaged veterans, Blatt employed this device to determine the kind and degree of language deficit. The test "... was developed primarily for use with adolescents and adults whose language abilities became impaired after normal language functioning was established."[13]

The test is divided into two main sections. They are:

1) Primarily Evaluative and Receptive Disturbances.

In this section are the items measuring visual, auditory and tactile agnosia, as well as Auditory Verbal Comprehension and Silent Reading Comprehension.

In the visual agnosia items, the subject is asked to identify a series of common objects, pictures of common objects, colors, forms, reduced size pictures, numbers, letters, printed words and printed sentences.

[10] J. Eisenson, *Examining for Aphasia, A Manual for the Examination of Aphasia and Related Disturbances.*

[11] H. Chenven, *Effects of Group Therapy Upon Language Recovery in Predominantly Expressive Aphasic Patients.*

[12] B. Blatt, *The Problem of Language Localization into Specific Brain Areas.*

[13] J. Eisenson, *op. cit.*, p. 29.

The auditory agnosia section includes items on the recognition of sounds and word identification.

The section on tactile agnosia involves items that test for object identification.

The Auditory Verbal Comprehension section includes a series of ten simple questions presented orally with four multiple choice answers. It is followed by the reading of four paragraphs with questions to be answered.

The Silent Reading Comprehension includes a series of ten simple questions and four multiple choice answers.

2) Predominantly Productive and Expressive Disturbances.

The Apraxias come under this section. The Non-verbal Apraxias section includes body parts, simple skills and pretended actions. The section on Verbal Apraxias tests for numbers, words and sentences. The aphasias include automatic speech, writing numbers and letters, spelling, writing from dictation, naming of body parts, word-finding, arithmetic computations and problems, clock setting and oral reading.

Eisenson employed standardized achievement test material whenever it was practicable. In explaining the design of the test, he points out:

> The items of information sought in the examination are intended to reveal. both the assets and deficits of the subject at the time of the examination.[14]

The administration of the test followed the directions recommended by Eisenson.

The scoring system was based upon a method of quantification whereby each correct response received a score of one and each failure a score of zero. The maximum potential score is 414.

Rationale for the Use of Performance Tests with Brain-damaged Subjects

The use of performance tests alone as evaluative devices has been reported in the literature on numerous occasions. Goldstein and

[14] *Loc. cit.*

Scheerer pointed out that "... the objective of the routine performance test is to determine the *actual* capacity of a subject which may not express itself in the same clear-cut manner on a verbal test."[15] In certain pathological cases, they believed that performance tests were "... especially superior to verbal tests."[16]

Wechsler stated: "It would clearly be unfair to use a combined Verbal and Performance Scale on subjects suffering from motor or visual defects or some special language handicap."[17] He thought that the Scale to employ with such subjects should be the one that does not penalize them for their disability. He stated that: "With such subjects it is often better to use one rather than another type of intelligence scale."[18]

Many investigators working with brain-damaged subjects have developed and employed specially constructed tests that they believed to be logical and appropriate to the task under consideration. Bauer[19] employed performance tests developed by students and faculty members as well as tests he developed personally and some published standarized tests in his investigation of a brain-damaged population of aphasics and non-aphasics.

Thurstone's findings motivated him to point out that his data "... indicate the desirability of not taking too seriously the differentiation between complex verbal tasks and perceptual tasks."[20] He believed that perceptual tasks may be a more effective way of evaluating reasoning than the complex verbal reasoning tasks.[21]

Indicating that no comprehensive theory of thinking or adequate definition of intelligence ever had been developed, Guilford stated: "Enough of the intellectual factors are known to suggest strongly the outlines of a system."[22] This he proceeded to do and found that an inspection of the list of about forty different known

15 K. Goldstein and M. Scheerer, *op. cit.*, p. 10.
16 *Loc. cit.*
17 D. Wechsler, *Measurement of Adult Intelligence*, p. 138.
18 *Loc. cit.*
19 R. W. Bauer and D. M. Becka, "Intellect after Cerebrovascular Accident".
20 L. L. Thurstone, *A Factorial Study of Perception*, p. 119.
21 *Ibid.*, pp. 111-112.
22 J. P. Guilford, "The Structure of Intellect", p. 267.

factors showed that the intellectual factors fell into two major groups. The great majority of them were thinking factors and the remainder were memory factors. He pointed out that: "For some time we have been aware that thinking factors tend to pair off according to the material or content used in the tests. For each factor of a certain kind found in verbal tests, there seems to be a mate found in tests composed of figures and designs."[23]

The Goldstein-Scheerer Cube Test[24]

This test is similar to the Kohs Block Design Test. It employs the same kind of blocks used in the Kohs test and the Block Designs subtest of the Wechsler-Bellevue Intelligence Scale Form I. There are four identical cubes with colored sides. Each of four sides of the cube bear one of the following colors: red, white, blue and yellow. Each of the two remaining sides bears two colors divided diagonally; one blue and yellow and the other red and white. There are two booklets containing twelve designs that are to be copied with the cubes. For each one of the twelve designs, there are six steps representing simplifications of the original design. These steps are graduated aids to facilitate the copying of the model. The purpose of these aids is to assist the normal subject "... in acquiring insight into the demands of the task and in learning to apply them to other phases of the test."[25]

Goldstein and Scheerer pointed out that in order to reproduce the design, two types of approach are possible, a concrete and an abstract. They stated:

> There is definite indication of impairment of abstract behavior if a subject cannot profit by the facilitating modifications, so that he fails again on the standard design.[26]

They continued:

[23] *Ibid.*, p. 269.
[24] K. Goldstein and M. Scheerer, *Abstract and Concrete Behavior; An Experimental Study with Special Tests.*
[25] *Ibid.*, p. 49.
[26] *Ibid.*, p. 56.

... whether or not a patient ever learns is a reasonable measure of the degree of disturbance. Any learning that occurs is a symptom of a lesser degree of deterioration. There is definite evidence that patients who improve in their mental status (e.g., after hemorrhages or operated brain tumors) also show improvement in their performance on this test.[27]

Since the test contains some designs that are presented on the horizontal base while other designs are presented on an angle, the ability to shift from one approach to another reflects the flexibility of the patient. Rigidity or flexibility is indicated also by the degree of perseverations of shape or color on the various designs or steps of a single design. Goldstein and Scheerer believed that this test enables the examiner to evaluate a subject's flexibility and "... determine whether a patient can or cannot assume the abstract attitude."[28]

The authors could not as yet evolve experimentally verifiable criteria for different levels of abstract and concrete behavior. However, the experimental findings in this test suggest that there are *degrees* of lesser and stronger concreteness in a subject, which correspondingly require more or less concrete aids.[29]

They concluded:

The test therefore should be suitable for studying impairment of abstract behavior in cases of mental deficiency due to abnormal development, brain lesions, dementia praecox.[30]

The test was administered according to the directions provided by Goldstein and Scheerer.

The scoring system was based upon a method developed by Boyd who used this test in a study concerned with the measurement of organic deterioration. After pointing out the merits and uses of the other Goldstein-Scheerer tests, he stated that "... the Cube test has finer discriminatory values among organic patients and is more susceptible to quantitative analysis."[31] Boyd suggested a decreasing

[27] *Loc. Cit.*
[28] *Ibid.*, p. 30.
[29] *Ibid.*, p. 57.
[30] *Loc. cit.*
[31] F. Boyd, "A Provisional Quantitative Scoring with Preliminary Norms for the Goldstein Scheerer Cube Test", pp. 148-153.

scale of points for each of the six steps, allowing points for a satisfactory performance as well as a satisfactory explanation. If a subject gives a satisfactory performance and explanation on Step I, he receives the maximum of ten points, that is, five points for a satisfactory explanation and five points for a satisfactory performance, and goes on to the next design. If the subject fails on the performance or explanation or both, he receives partial or no credit and goes on to the next facilitating step. No credit is given, however, unless the subject is able to complete the design from the card of Step I.

Table III indicates the possible score at each of the facilitating steps for a given design. The maximum potential score is 120.

To measure adaptive flexibility, a score of one point was given for each production that repeated some aspect, whether shape, position, color or pattern of the design immediately preceding it, and thereby caused the response to be incorrect.

TABLE III

A Quantification of the Goldstein Scheerer Cube Test

Step	I	II	III	IV	V	VI
Performance	5.	2.5	2	1.5	1.	.5
Explanation	5.	2.5	2	1.5	1.	.5
Performance and Explanation	10.	5.	4.	3.	2.	1.

The Goldstein-Scheerer Stick Test[32]

The purpose of this test is to determine whether the subject is able to copy figures composed of sticks and reproduce them from memory.

The test material consists of the following sticks: four 4″ sticks, twelve 3″ sticks, eight 2″ sticks and six $\frac{3}{4}$″ sticks. All the sticks are made of an ivory colored plastic material.

The test is divided into two parts. In the first section, the Copy

[32] K. Goldstein and M. Scheerer, *op. cit.*, pp. 131-149.

section, the examiner constructs a geometric figure with the sticks. The subject is asked to make a copy while looking at the sample figure. There are 36 stimulus figures. The sequence in which these figures are given represents a scale of increasingly intricate configurations in the geometrical and numerical sense. In the second section, the Reproduction section, the examiner constructs and presents the same 36 stimulus figures to the subject in the same sequence. In this instance, however, after the examiner constructs the figure with the sticks, he has the subject study the figure for 5 to 10 seconds and then removes the figure. The subject is required to reproduce the figure from memory. In both sections, the examiner constructs the stimulus figure outside the view of the subject.

On the Reproduction section, the exposure time was five seconds on models numbered one through fourteen and ten seconds on the remaining models.

The administration of the test was according to the directions provided by Goldstein and Scheerer.[33]

In analyzing the designs on this test, Goldstein and Scheerer stated:

> They are mere configurations of spatial direction in a detached purified sense. They imply both space and direction as entities in themselves. Therefore, they are abstract features in an abstract geometrical space; bearing no reference to a tangible life situation.[34]

They believed that "To reproduce the purely *geometric* figures, the normal subject has to combine *both* attitudes, the concrete and the abstract."[35] They pointed out that while the normal person is not aware of it "The copying or reproducing of senseless figures requires the abstract attitude."[36]

The test was scored by giving one point for each of the following criteria: (a) the correct number of sticks, (b) the correct shape, (c) the correct position or direction, (d) the correct size of sticks, and

[33] *Ibid.*, pp. 131, 148-149.

[34] *Ibid.*, p. 131.

[35] *Loc. cit.*

[36] *Ibid.*, p. 133.

(e) the correct area between sticks. The maximum potential score is 157 for each of the two section of the test.

Since the degree of flexibility or rigidity was reflected by the number of perseverations of designs, adaptive flexibility was determined for this test. A score of one point was given for each production on both sections of the test that repeated some aspect of the design immediately preceding it and thereby caused the response to be incorrect. The repetition could be in any one or all of the five scorable areas indicated previously.

A memory score was determined for each subject by calculating the total score on the Reproduction section of this test.

The Wechsler Bellevue Intelligence Scale Form I (Performance Section)[37]

Only the Performance section of this test was administered to each subject since the primary concern of this research was with non-verbal intellectual functioning.

The Performance section consists of five subtests, each of which has time limits. The subtests are:

1. *Picture Arrangement Test.* This test consists of seven series of cards. Each one of the series are made up of pictures, which, when placed in a correct sequence, tell a story. The cartoon-like pictures "... are presented to the subject in a disarranged order and he is asked to put them together in the right order so that they make a sensible story".[38] The first series is a sample set used to demonstrate the task. The time limit for the first three items is one minute each, and for the remaining three items two minutes each. For the last two series additional credits are given for satisfactory arrangements within various time limits. The maximum potential score is 21.

2. *Picture Completion Test.* In this test, the subject is required "... to discover and name the missing part of an incompletely drawn

[37] D. Wechsler, *The Measurement of Adult Intelligence.*
[38] *Ibid.*, p. 87.

picture".[39] There are fifteen cards with pictures on them which are presented to the subject in numerical order. Each card is exposed for the maximum time of 20 seconds. The maximum potential score is 15.

3. *Block Design Test.* This test consists of sixteen cubes and nine designs, the first two of which are samples that are used by the examiner for demonstration purposes. The blocks are similar to those used in the Kohs Block Test. The first five designs require four cubes, the next two designs require nine cubes and the last design employs all sixteen cubes. The maximum potential score is 42.

4. *Object Assembly Test.* This test consists of three separate figure formboards — a *Manikin*, a *Feature Profile* and a *Hand*. These figures are divided into several pieces like a jigsaw puzzle. The Manikin consists of six pieces, the others of seven pieces each. The subject is required to put these pieces together into the correct configuration.[40] The time limit is two minutes on the first item and three minutes on the other items. The maximum potential score is 26.

5. *Digit Symbol Test.* This test requires the association of certain symbols with numbers. After a demonstration by the examiner, the subject has to fill in, with a pencil, as many blank squares as he can with the correct symbol that belongs with a given number the time limit is ninty seconds. The maximum potential score is 67.

For the purpose of scoring this test, the raw scores achieved on each subtest were used. It was believed that the raw scores more sharply delineated the achievement level of the subject since a weighted score often represented two or more raw score points. The raw scores for each subtest are provided in the test manual.[41]

Essentially, the Picture Arrangement Test involves visual organization, planning ability and anticipatory thinking, as well as social comprehension. The Picture Completion Test requires visual

[39] *Ibid.*, p. 90.
[40] *Ibid.*, p. 96.
[41] *Ibid.*, pp. 171-185.

organization, concentration on visual material and recognition of relevant details. The Block Design Test requires the ability to analyze a pattern or differentiate it into parts and then synthesize the pattern by reproducing it. The task, like the Object Assembly and Digit Symbol Tests, involves visual organization. In the Object Assembly Test, the visual organization involves the recognition of patterns or the ability to grasp whole pattern by means of anticipation from its more or less meaningful parts. The Digit Symbol Test, in addition, involves motor set and psychomotor speed.

The Bender Visual Motor Gestalt Test[42]

This test consists of nine simple designs each of which is presented to a subject (in a standardized numerical order) on individual 4 × 6 white cards for him to copy on a standard sheet of $8\frac{1}{2}'' \times 11''$ white paper. These geometric figures were selected by Bender, from many designs originally used by Wertheimer, and incorporated into a test for clinical use and to study gestalt function. Bender stated:

> The gestalt function may be defined as that function of the integrated organism whereby it responds to a given constellation of stimuli as a whole; the response itself being a constellation, or pattern, or gestalt. All integrative processes within the nervous system occur in constellations, or patterns or gestalten.[43]

Bender went on to say:

> The final gestalt is therefore, composed of the original pattern in space (visual pattern), the temporal factor of becoming and the personal-sensory-motor factor. ... This pattern of action may be expected to vary in different maturation or growth levels and in pathological states, organically or functionally determined.[44]

The test has been widely used in a variety of investigations. There have been studies to estimate maturation, intelligence, psychological disturbances, the effect of injury to the cortex and to follow the effects of convulsive therapy.

[42] L. Bender, *A Visual Motor Gestalt Test and Its Clinical Use.*
[43] *Ibid.*, p. 3.
[44] *Ibid.*, p. 5.

In a study employing the Bender Gestalt Test, Pascal and Suttell supported Bender's position. They reported that "Adults of normal intelligence without known cortical damage do not, in our experience, fail to reproduce the essential Gestalten."[45] Their findings indicated that:

> Reproductions resulting in fragmentation, destruction, or primitivation of the Gestalten are regularly obtained from children below the age of six, from patients immediately after convulsive therapy, from brain-damaged individuals, paretics, and seniles; in other words, wherever there is a cortical deficit or damage.[46]

The instructions and procedure recommended by Pascal and Suttell have been employed in the administration and scoring of this test. There are 105 deviations from the test stimulus that are given different values by these authors depending on the frequency of occurrence in the population they studied. Table IV lists the criteria for scoring developed by Pascal and Suttell. It indicates the type of deviation and the points assigned to it, for each of the eight numbered designs as well as several deviations in the over-all configuration design and the points for each. Design A is not scored individually. The subject's score is the total raw score achieved for the test.

Pascal and Suttell stated:

> The evidence is, we think, sufficiently clear so that we may make the statement that the greater the damge to the cortex through convulsive therapy, amentia, lack of maturation, trauma, etc., the greater the deviations from the stimulus, and on our scoring system the higher the score on the B-G test.[47]

While they found that the Bender Gestalt scores were not a function of sex or affected much by drawing ability, they did conclude that "There is little doubt in our minds that Bender Gestalt performance is correlated with I.Q."[48]

[45] G. R. Pascal and B. J. Suttell, *The Bender Gestalt Test*, p. 8.
[46] *Loc. cit.*
[47] *Ibid.*, p. 9.
[48] *Ibid.*, p. 22.

TABLE IV

Scoring Criteria Bender-Gestalt Test[49] *(Based on Pascal & Suttell)*

Criteria	Score	Design Number
1. Wavy line	2	1,2
2. Dots, dashes and circles	3	1,3,5
3. Dashes	2	1,3,5
4. Circles	8	1,3,5
5. Number of dots	2 each	1,3,5
6. Dashes or dots	3	2
7. Shape of Circle	3	2
8. Cir. Miss. Ext.	3	2
9. Circle touching	5	2
10. Double row	8	1
11. Extra row	8	3
12. Dev. slant	3	2
13. Workover	2	1,2,3,5,6,8
14. Sec. attempt	3 each	1,2,3,4,5,6,7,8
15. Rotation	8	1,2,3,4,5,6,7,8
16. Design Missing	8	1,2,3,4,5,6,7,8
17. No. of Columns	2 each	2,
18. Fig. on 2 lines	8	2
19. Guide lines	2	2,3,4,5,6,7,8
20. Asymmetry	3	3,5,6
21. Asymmetrical Crv.	3	4
22. Blunting	8	3
23. Distortion	8	3,4,5,6,7,8
24. Break Curve	4	4
25. Curve not center	1	4
26. Curls	4	4
27. Not joined	8	4
28. Curve rotation	3	4
29. Touch-up	8	4,6
30. Tremor	4	4,,6,7,8
31. Ext. join dot	3	5
32. Ext. rotation	3	5
33. Angles	3	6
34. Pt. crossing	2 each	6
35. Curve extra	8	6
36. Double line	1 each	6,7,8
37. Ends not joined	8	7,8
38. Angles Ext.	3	7,8
39. Angles Miss.	3	7,8
40. Ext. scat.	3	7,8
41. Pace. Des. A.	2	Configuration Design
42. Overlap	2 each	Configuration Design
43. Compression	3	Configuration Design
44. Lines Drawn	8	Configuration Design
45. Order	2	Configuration Design
46. No order	8	Configuration Design
47. Rel. size	8	Configuration Design

[49] Pascal and Suttell, *op. cit.*

In a study of 142 mildly retarded adults, Taylor employed the Bender Gestalt test and the scoring system of Pascal and Suttell. He compared the results with that of the Wechsler Adult Intelligence Scale and concluded, "In short, it has been shown that the BG (Bender Gestalt) can be viewed as a valid test of performance intelligence."[50]

TREATMENT OF DATA

Subproblem 1. To determine the extent of language facility and non-verbal intellectual functioning in hemiplegic patients with aphasia.

To describe the central tendency and variability of this group in each test, the mean, standard deviation, and standard error of the mean were calculated. The formula employed to compute the mean is:

a)

$$\bar{X} = \frac{\Sigma x}{N}$$

where $\bar{X}$ stands for the mean, x equals the test score and N stands for the number of subjects.[51]

For the computation of the standard deviation, the formula used was:

$$s = \sqrt{\frac{N\Sigma X^2 - (\Sigma X)^2}{N(N-1)}}$$

in which s stands for the standard deviation, X equals the deviation from the mean and N represents the size of the sample.[52]

The standard error of the mean was computed by using the formula:

$$s\bar{x} = \frac{s}{\sqrt{N}}$$

[50] James B. Taylor, "The Bender Gestalt as a Measure of Intelligence and Adjustment in the Lower Intellectual Range", p. 595.

[51] H. M. Walker and J. Lev, *Elementary Statistical Methods*, p. 88.

[52] *Ibid.*, p. 89.

where $s_{\bar{x}}$ equals the standard error of the mean, s stands for the standard deviation and N equals the number of cases.[53]

As a further description of the Aphasic group, 21 product-moment correlation co-efficients were computed to determine the relationship between each combination of tests. The computational formula used was:

$$r = \frac{\Sigma xy - \frac{(\Sigma x)(\Sigma y)}{N}}{\sqrt{(\Sigma x^2 - \frac{\Sigma x^2}{N})\ (\Sigma y^2 - \frac{\Sigma y^2}{N})}}$$

where r stands for the correlation co-efficient, X equals the score for test one and Y equals the score for test two, N equals the number of pairs.[54]

Edwards[55] Table VI was used to determine if any of the 21 r's are significantly different from zero. With thirteen degrees of freedom, r must equal or exceed 0.514 to be significantly different from zero.

Subproblem 2. To determine the extent of language facility and non-verbal intellectual functioning in hemiplegic patients without aphasia.

The same statistical procedures were applied to the group of hemiplegic patients without aphasia as were employed with the Aphasic group in subproblem 1.

Subproblem 3. To make intra- and inter- group comparisons of the two research populations on the basis of the data obtained in subproblems 1 and 2.

In order to compare the two groups on the basis of the variables to be measured, a t-test was applied to each of the seven pairs of means to determine the significance of their differences. The test employed was for small independent samples. The computational formula used was:

53 *Ibid.*, p. 213.
54 A. L. Edwards, *Statistical Methods for the Behavioral Sciences*, p. 147.
55 *Ibid.*, p. 502.

$$t = \frac{\bar{X}_1 - \bar{X}_2}{S\bar{x}_1 - \bar{x}_2}$$

where $$S\bar{x}_1 - \bar{x}_2 = \sqrt{\left(\frac{\Sigma x_1^2 + \Sigma x_2^2}{N_1 + N_2 - 2}\right)\left(\frac{1}{N_1} + \frac{1}{N_2}\right)}$$

and where $$\Sigma X_1^2 = \Sigma x_1^2 - \frac{(\Sigma X_1)^2}{N_1}$$

In this formula, $\bar{x}_1$ stands for the mean of the Aphasic group, $\bar{x}_2$ stands for the mean of the Non-aphasic group, and N_1 equals the number of cases in the Aphasic group, N_2 equals the number of cases in the Non-aphasic group.[56]

Since the experimental hypothesis in this study is the null hypothesis, the test for significance is a two-tailed one and consequently becomes less influenced by skewness. It was evaluated, based upon Fisher's special table for *t*, at the five per cent level of confidence with $N_1 + N_2 - 2 = 28$ degrees of freedom.

Boneau has shown that only extreme deviations from normality or homogeneity of variance, even with small samples, produce erroneous points of significance.[57] Since homogeneity of variance is an assumption underlying the *t*-test, and since it would be interesting to note whether one group was more variable than the other on one or more of the seven tests, the *F*-test was applied to each of the seven pairs of variances (S^2) as determined in subproblems one and two. The F-ratio was established by placing the larger variance over the smaller for each pair so that

$$F = \frac{S_1^2}{S_2^2}$$

Where variance S^2 equals (standard deviation)^2, S_1 stands for that group with the highest variance on a particular test and S_2 stands for the group with the lowest variance on the same particular test.

The obtained F was then evaluated with $(N_1 - 1)$ and $(N_2 - 1)$ degrees of freedom at the five per cent level confidence.[58]

[56] *Ibid.*, p. 253.

[57] Alan Boneau, "The Effects of Violation of Assumptions Underlying the *t*-test", pp. 43-64.

[58] A. L. Edwards, *op. cit.*, pp. 490-499.

4. TREATMENT OF THE DATA

In the following sections, a quantitative and qualitative analysis of the obtained data is presented. The statistical techniques employed were described in Chapter III, pp. 58-60.

QUANTITATIVE ANALYSIS

Certain specific problems were stated in this study. The first specific problem was:

To determine the extent of language facility and non-verbal intellectual functioning in hemiplegic patients with aphasia. This group is designated the Aphasic group.

To determine language facility, the Eisenson Test for Aphasia was administered to each subject. The Goldstein-Scheerer Cube Test, the Goldstein-Scheerer Stick Test, the Wechsler-Bellevue Intelligence Scale Form I (Performance Section), and the Bender Visual Motor Gestalt Test were administered to each subject to determine non-verbal intellectual functioning and adaptive flexibility.

In order to evaluate the results of these various tests, for the Aphasic group, as indicated in Specific Problem Number One, the mean, standard deviation and standard error of the mean were calculated for each of the variables.

Table V presents the results obtained for the Aphasic group on each of the tests.

(The Test titles in Table V will hold for each Table VI through IX)

On the Eisenson Test, the Aphasic mean score is 137.33 with a standard deviation of 71.81 and a standard error of 18.56.

The mean score for the Aphasic group on the Goldstein-Scheerer

TABLE V

Means, Sigmas, and Standard Error of Means of Fifteen Aphasic Patients on Various Tests and on Flexibility

Test	Mean	Sigma	Standard Error of Means
1) Eisenson[a]	137.33	71.81	18.56
2) Cube[b]	71.43	35.19	9.09
3) Stick Copy[c]	145.80	15.28	3.95
4) Stick Reproduction[d]	134.53	23.33	6.02
5) Wechsler[e]	38.13	23.97	6.19
6) Bender[f]	74.20	36.20	9.35
7) Flexibility[g]	20.93	24.47	5.29

[a] The Eisenson Test for Aphasia; [b] The Goldstein-Scheerer Cube Test; [c] The Goldstein-Scheerer Stick Test (Copy Section); [d] The Goldstein-Scheerer Stick Test (Reproduction Section); [e] The Wechsler Bellevue Intelligence Scale Form I (Performance Section); [f] The Bender Gestalt Test; [g] Adaptive Flexibility.

Cube Test is 71.43 with a standard deviation of 35.19 and a standard error of 9.09.

For the Goldstein-Scheerer Stick Test (Copy Section), the Aphasic mean score is 145.80, the standard deviation 15.28 and the standard error 3.95.

On the Goldstein-Scheerer Stick Test (Reproduction Section) the Aphasic group mean score is 134.53, the standard deviation is 23.33 and the standard error is 6.02.

The Aphasic group mean score on the Wechsler Bellevue Intelligence Scale (Performance Section), is 38.13, the standard deviation 23.97, and the standard error 6.19.

On the Bender Visual Motor Gestalt Test, the Aphasic group mean score is 74.20, with a standard deviation of 36.20 and a standard error of 9.35.

For the Aphasic group, the mean Flexibility score is 20.93, with a standard deviation of 24.47, and a standard error of 5.29.

To determine the relationship between each combination of tests, for the Aphasic group, twenty-one product-moment correlation coefficients were computed.

Table VI presents the intertest correlation coefficients.

With 13 degrees of freedom, an r must equal or exceed 0.514 to be significantly different from zero, at the .05 level of confidence.

The Eisenson Test shows low, but statistically non-significant, correlations with each of the non-verbal performance tests of intellectual functioning. The correlations of the Eisenson Test, with the Cube of .12, with the Stick Copy of .09, with the Stick Reproduction of .21, with the Wechsler of .19, with the Bender of .24, and with Flexibility of .15, are not statistically significant at the .05 level of confidence.

The intertest correlation of all of the non-verbal performance tests of intellectual functioning are statistically significant at the .05 level of confidence.

TABLE VI

Correlation Coefficients of Various Tests for a Group of Fifteen Aphasic Patients

Eisenson	Cube	Stick Copy	Stick Reproduction	Wechsler	Bender	Flexibility
1) Eisenson	.12	.09	.21	.19	.24	.15
2) Cube	—	.64*	.73*	.83*	.69	.65*
3) Stick Copy		—	.87*	.64*	.72*	.78*
4) Stick Reproduction			—	.66*	.66*	.83*
5) Wechsler				—	.63*	.58*
6) Bender					—	.59*
7) Flexibility						—

* = Significant Correlations at the .05 level of confidence.

The Cube Test correlations of .64 with the Stick Copy, of .73 with the Stick Reproduction, of .83 with the Wechsler, of .69 with the Bender, and of .65 with Flexibility, are all statistically significant at the .05 level of confidence.

The Stick Copy r's of .87 with the Stick Reproduction, .64 with the Wechsler, .72 with the Bender, and .78 with Flexibility, are all statistically significant at the .05 level of confidence.

The Stick Reproduction correlation with the Wechsler is .66, with the Bender .66, and with Flexibility, .83. All the correlations are statistically significant at the .05 level of confidence.

The Wechsler *r*'s of .63 with the Bender and .58 with Flexibility are statistically significant at the .05 level of confidence.

The Bender *r* of .59 with Flexibility is statistically significant at the .05 level.

The second specific problem in this study was:

To determine the extent of language facility and non-verbal intellectual functioning in hemiplegic patients without aphasia. This group is designated the Non-aphasic Group.

The same battery of tests administered to the Aphasic group (p. 61) to determine language facility and non-verbal intellectual functioning was employed with the Non-aphasic group for the same purpose.

The results of these various tests were evaluated for the Non-aphasic group, as indicated in Specific Problem Number Two, by calculating a mean, standard deviation and standard error of the mean for each of the variables.

Table VII presents the results obtained for the Non-aphasic group on each of the variables.

The mean score for the Non-aphasic group on the Eisenson Test is 387.33 with a standard deviation of 21.61 and a standard error of 5.58.

On the Goldstein-Scheerer Cube Test, the Non-aphasic group mean score is 47.37, the standard deviation 38.29, and the standard error 9.89.

The Goldstein-Scheerer Stick Test (Copy Section) mean score for the Non-aphasic group is 120.73, with a standard deviation of 35.53 and a standard error of 9.17.

For the Goldstein-Scheerer Stick Test (Reproduction Section) the Non-aphasic group mean score is 106.33, the standard deviation 30.91 and the standard error 7.98.

The Non-aphasic group mean score on the Wechsler Bellevue Intelligence Scale (Performance Section), is 33.55, the standard deviation 22.18 and the standard error 5.73.

TABLE VII

Means, Sigmas and Standard Error of the Means of Fifteen Non-Aphasic Patients on Various Tests and on Flexibility

Test	Mean	Sigma	Standard Error of Means
1) Eisenson	387.33	21.61	5.58
2) Cube	47.37	38.29	9.89
3) Stick Copy	120.73	35.53	9.17
4) Stick Reproduction	106.33	30.91	7.98
5) Wechsler	33.55	22.18	5.73
6) Bender	138.87	59.79	15.44
7) Flexibility	37.40	29.90	7.72

The mean score for the Non-aphasic group on the Bender Visual Motor Gestalt Test, is 138.87, with a standard deviation of 59.79 and a standard error of 15.44.

For Adaptive Flexibility, the Non-aphasic mean score, is 37.40, the standard deviation is 29.90 and the standard error is 7.72.

Twenty-one product-moment correlation coefficients were calculated to determine the relationship between each combination of tests for the Non-aphasic group.

With 13 degrees of freedom, an *r* must equal or exceed 0.514 to be significantly different from zero, at the .05 level of confidence.

TABLE VIII

Correlation Coefficients of Various Tests for a Group of Fifteen Non-aphasic Patients

	Eisenson	Cube	Stick Copy	Stick Reproduction	Wechsler	Bender	Flexibility
1) Eisenson	—	.10	.49	.38	.30	.48	.29
2) Cube		—	.75*	.78*	.85*	.72*	.55*
3) Copy			—	.94*	.72*	.86*	.76*
4) Reproduction				—	.74*	.76*	.85*
5) Wechsler					—	.76*	.52*
6) Bender						—	.57*
7) Flexibility							—

* = Significant Correlations at the .05 level of confidence.

Table VIII shows the results for all the combination of tests for the Non-aphasic Group.

Although the Eisenson Test shows low correlations with the non-verbal performance tests of intellectual functioning, none of these are statistically significant. The Eisenson Test correlation of .10 with the Cube Test, .49 with the Stick Copy, .38 with the Stick Reproduction, .30 with the Wechsler, .48 with the Bender and .29 with Flexibility, are not statistically significant at the .05 level of confidence.

For all of the non-verbal performance tests of intellectual functioning for the Non-aphasic Group, the intertest correlations are statistically significant at the .05 level of confidence.

The Cube Test correlations of .75 with the Stick Copy, of .78 with the Stick Reproduction, of .85 with the Wechsler, of .72 with the Bender and .55 with Flexibility, are all statistically significant at the .05 level of confidence.

The Stick Copy correlations of .94 with the Stick Reproduction, of .72 with the Wechsler, of .86 with the Bender and .76 with Flexibility, are all statistically significant at the .05 level of confidence.

The Stick Reproduction correlations of .74 with the Wechsler, of .76 for the Bender and .85 with Flexibility, are statistically significant at the .05 level of confidence.

For the Wechsler, an *r* of .76 with the Bender and .52 with Flexibility are statistically significant at the .05 level of confidence.

An *r* of .57 for the Bender with Flexibility is significant statistically at the .05 level.

The third specific problem in this study was:

To make intra- and inter-group comparisons of the two research populations on the basis of the data obtained in subproblems one and two.

In order to determine the significance of the mean differences between the two groups, a *t*-test was applied to each of the seven pairs of means. Table IX presents the results obtained for each of the comparisons.

The *F*-test is applied to each of the seven pairs of variances as determined in Specific Problems Number One and Two, to determine whether one group was more variable than the other on one or more of the seven variables. The results are presented in Table IX.

Eisenson Test for Aphasia

The obtained t of 12.46 for the Eisenson Test is statistically significant beyond the .05 level of confidence. The hypothesis of sampling from the same population is rejected. It indicates that the Non-aphasic group is a sample from a population with a mean much higher than the mean of the population from which the Aphasic group is a sample. That is, the populations, as revealed by the Eisenson Test, are significantly different with the Non-aphasic group performing at a significantly higher level on the materials of the Eisenson Test. A description of this test is presented on pages 46-47.

On the basis of an F-ratio of 11.04, the hypothesis of equal variance is rejected. The variability of the Aphasic group on this test is significantly higher than that of the Non-aphasic group.

Goldstein-Scheerer Cube Test

As Table IX reveals, a t of 1.79 for the Goldstein-Scheerer Cube Test is not statistically significant at the .05 level of confidence. This indicates that there is no significant difference in performance between the two groups as revealed by the Cube Test.

An F of 1.18 is not statistically significant indicating no significant differences in variability between the Aphasic and Non-aphasic groups on the Cube Test. A description of this test is presented on pages 51-52.

Goldstein-Scheerer Stick Test (Copy Section)

For this test, a t of 2.51 is obtained, as Table IX shows, which is statistically significant at the .05 level. The indications are that the Aphasic group is functioning at a significantly higher level than the Non-aphasic group on this test.

TABLE IX

A Comparison of the Aphasic and the Non-Aphasic Groups on the Basis of Data Presented in Tables V and VII

Test	M_A [a]	M_{NA} [b]	$Sigma_A$ [c]	$Sigma_{NA}$ [d]	$S.E._A$ [e]	$S.E._{NA}$ [f]	Diff. [g] M	Diff. [h] Sigma	Diff. [i] S.E.	F [j]	t [k]
Eisenson	137.33	387.33	71.81	21.61	18.56	5.58	−250.00	50.20	12.98	11.04*	12.46*
Cube	71.43	47.37	35.19	38.29	9.09	9.89	24.06	−3.10	−.80	1.18	1.79
Stick Copy	145.80	120.73	15.78	35.53	3.95	9.17	25.07	20.25	−5.22	5.41*	2.51*
Stick Reproduction	134.53	106.33	23.33	30.91	6.02	7.98	28.20	−7.58	−.96	1.76	2.82*
Wechsler	38.13	33.55	23.97	22.18	6.19	5.73	4.58	1.79	.46	1.17	.54
Bender	74.20	138.87	36.20	59.79	9.35	15.44	−64.67	−23.59	−6.09	3.73*	3.58*
Flexibility	20.93	37.40	24.47	29.90	5.29	7.72	−16.47	−5.43	−1.43	2.18	1.76

[a] M_A = Aphasic Mean [b] Non-aphasic Mean; [c] Aphasic Standard deviation; [d] Non-aphasic Standard deviation; [e] Aphasic Standard Error; [f] Non-aphasic Standard Error; [g] $M_A - M_{NA}$; [h] $Sigma_A - Sigma_{NA}$; [i] $S.E._A - S.E._{NA}$; [j] For each F: d.f. = 14 and 14: $F.05 = 2.48$; [k] d.f. = 28: $t.05 = 2.048$.
* = Significant at the .05 level of confidence.

The obtained F of 5.41 is statistically significant at the .05 level and the hypothesis of equal variance is rejected. The Non-aphasic group demonstrates a significantly higher variability on this test than the Aphasic group. A description of this test is presented on pages 51-52.

Goldstein-Scheerer Stick Test (Reproduction Section)

A *t* of 2.82 is obtained for the Goldstein-Scheerer Stick Test (Reproduction Section). This is statistically significant at the .05 level of confidence indicating that the populations of the two groups, as measured by this test, are different with the Aphasic group performing on a significantly higher level.

The obtained *F* of 1.76 for this test is not statistically significant and the hypothesis of no significant difference in variability between the two groups is retained.

A description of this test is indicated on pages 51-52.

Wechsler Bellevue Intelligence Scale Form I (Performance Section)

For the Wechsler-Bellevue Intelligence Scale Form I (Performance Section), a *t* of .54 is obtained which is not statistically significant. It is indicated that there is no significant difference in the performance of the two groups as measured by this test and that aphasia is not a handicapping condition on this kind of material.

An *F* of 1.17 is not statistically significant for this test, indicating that there is no significant difference in variability between the two groups.

A description of this test is presented on pages 53-55.

Bender Visual Motor Gestalt Test

On the Bender Visual Motor Gestalt Test, the higher the score, the lower is the quality of the performance. The obtained *t* of 3.58 is significant statistically at the .05 level of confidence, indicating that the two populations, as measured by this test, are different with the Aphasic group demonstrating significant superiority over the Non-aphasic group.

The obtained F of 3.73 is statistically significant at the .05 level of confidence. It is concluded that the hypothesis of equal variance is rejected. The Non-aphasic group is significantly more variable than the Aphasic group on this test.

A description of the Bender Test is presented on pages 55-56.

Adaptive Flexibility

Table IX (p. 68), reveals a t of 1.76 for *Adaptive Flexibility*. This is not statistically significant at the .05 level of confidence, indicating that there is no significant difference in the population of both groups as measured by this test.

An F of 2.18, as shown in Table IX is not statistically significant at the .05 level and the hypothesis of equal variance for both groups is retained.

The Adaptive Flexibility score is the sum total of all the instances of perseveration on the Cube, the Stick Copy, and the Stick Reproduction Tests. Therefore, the higher the score on this variable, the lower the demonstrated ability to shift and the more rigidity indicated.

QUALITATIVE ANALYSIS

Comprehension of Instructions

Many of the subjects in this study demonstrated some difficulty in comprehending the instructions given for one or more of the tests. While this was true for subjects in both groups, it was most true for the Aphasic group where all but one, Subject #8, exhibited this difficulty. Seven non-aphasics demonstrated this difficulty.

Subject #19 achieved the highest score in the Non-aphasic group on the Cube Test. However, on Design I, which is a one-color design, he said: "I don't quite get that. That's only one." The examiner repeated the instructions. The subject consistently got the design correct on each facilitating step but reverted to a single cube on Step I. On Step Ia, he made the design with 4 blocks but said: "That would be a single one, wouldn't it? Well, I would take it as a single." He pushed away 3 cubes and left one. He failed Design I because of this uncertainty about the size. However, on Design VI, which is a one-color design also, he demonstrated no difficulty with size and succeeded on the initial presentation.

An aphasic, Subject #3, had much difficulty in understanding the instructions at the beginning of the Cube Test. After the third facilitating step of Design I, the examiner repeated the instructions. The patient said: "Oh", and successfully completed the design quickly. She went on to achieve full or partial scores on each of the first six designs. That she had learned something on Design I was demonstrated by the facility with which she succeeded on Design VI. The difficulty with size which she had exhibited on Design I was not present on Design VI.

A non-aphasic, Subject #24, after the third item on the Stick Copy Test, stopped and complained: "I don't quite understand what you want me to do." This same subject on Design I of the Cube Test asked: "Can I make it with one?" In both instances, when the instructions were repeated, she was able to succeed on the designs.

Subject #14, an aphasic, had extreme difficulty in understanding the instructions on the Stick Copy Test, although the examiner repeated them many times. For the first 4 figures on the test where only one stick was employed, the patient merely gestured with his finger. The examiner pointed to the pile of sticks and the patient picked one and held it in his hand. The examiner indicated that it should be placed on the table, which the patient did, and succeeded on the items.

Another aphasic, Subject #11, did not understand the instructions despite several repetitions. Finally the examiner demonstrated that he was to place the sticks together to form a figure. The subject was then able to do the entire test receiving a score of 151 out of a possible 157.

The same difficulty in comprehension of instructions was demonstrated on the Wechsler Bellevue by several subjects in both groups. A non-aphasic, Subject #30, tried to make the cards meet flush on the Picture Arrangement subtest. An aphasic, Subject #6, could not understand what was demanded of him on this same subtest and repeated several times: "I don't know what da hell."

The Bender Gestalt Test did not present as great a problem in this regard although one aphasic, Subject #3, did nothing after looking at Card I. When the instructions were repeated, she expressed surprise that she was expected to copy *dots*. Another subject wanted to copy the figures on the card rather than on the paper.

Behavioral Observations

During the testing, certain behavioral manifestations were noted that have been reported in the literature, as frequently observed in brain-damaged subjects. An analysis is made of only that behavior which was overtly exhibited by the subjects. Certain interesting group differences are revealed. It should be noted that for most of the subjects, these characteristics became apparent as the nature of the task became more difficult for them to perform successfully. Once these psychological and emotional factors are present, they tend to interfere with the effective functioning of the individual. In some cases, these two factors tend to be so disruptive that it becomes difficult to determine how much of the deficit in functioning is due to the brain lesion and how much to the psychological and emotional overlay.

Lability. — While no non-aphasic demonstrated lability, five aphasics did. Only one, Subject #15, became so agitated that the testing was halted for the day. This occurred during the administration of the Stick Reproduction Test. On figure #11, the patient appeared annoyed and depressed after three perseverations. "They're all the same. That's not way it was but — (waves hand). That's third or fourth time I did it like that." He failed the following three items and he became more agitated. On figure #15, he began to laugh hysterically and said many times: "I don't want to do it no more. I'm pulled up with it." He made #15 incorrectly, but corrected it saying: "This should be this way". He then said: "I don't want to do this anymore. This is nothin'." The session was ended.

In another instance, a very depressed aphasic, Subject #4, became quite frustrated when he was unable to state his birthday. Tears came to his eyes and he struck his right hand in disgust. After the session, he kissed his left hand and again struck his right hand.

Hostility and Anger. — Nine non-aphasics overtly expressed anger or hostility towards the examiner, the test, themselves, or others. Only four aphasics did the same. Although many subjects appeared somewhat depressed, 7 aphasics overtly demonstrated marked depression by sighing, crying, or verbalizing it. Only one non-aphasic manifested similar symptoms.

Feelings of Inadequacy. — Many subjects, in both groups, expressed feelings of inadequacy in one way or another. The Aphasic group tended to blame themselves for their inability to perform a task, usually saying: "I don't know." "I can't do that." or by making some self-derogating remark. While this was true for the Non-aphasic group also, they often blamed the situation or the test material, saying: "I don't think I can do it. I think it's my teeth, that's why." or "It don't make it. It should, but it don't." or "It can't be done with only 4 blocks."

Level of Aspiration. — Most subjects, in both groups, demonstrated a strong desire and effort to achieve on these tests and to gain the approval of the examiner. Subject #7 worked so hard trying to recall information, he began breathing very heavily, making panting sounds. Subject #25 worked very rapidly and leaned back in his chair with great satisfaction when he completed a task successfully. Although some subjects verbalized or indicated a desire to quit when they found a task too difficult, they continued working with a little encouragement from the examiner. Very often, subjects would ask for the examiner's approval after completing a task or seek such approval by acting in an ingratiating manner.

5. DISCUSSION

BASIC HYPOTHESIS

It was hypothesized that no consistent relationship exists between ability to engage in non-verbal intellectual tasks and language disturbance. This hypothesis has been sustained. While the Non-aphasic group demonstrates significant superiority over the Aphasic group on the test of language ability, it does not demonstrate a similar superiority on the non-verbal performance tests of intellectual ability.

Test Battery

The selection of the tests for this study was based upon a careful consideration of the nature of the investigation and the population involved in this research. The rationale for the use of performance tests has been indicated on pages 47-49. The final choice was a battery consisting of tests commonly employed with brain-damaged subjects in institutions as well as in research in order to evaluate their level of language and intellectual functioning. The devices selected have been used by the researcher for several years as part of a regular battery of tests to evaluate the level of intellectual functioning of brain-damaged patients.

Eisenson Test for Aphasia. — This test is the instrument regularly used at the institutions where this research was done for the purpose of determining the level of language ability of a subject as well as the nature of any language disability.

The Eisenson Test clearly delineates the two groups in terms of language ability. Tables V (page 62) and VII (page 65) indicate that the Non-aphasic group demonstrates superiority over the Aphasic group in the area of language. A t of 12.46, as shown in Table IX (page 68), is significant statistically beyond the .05 level of confidence established for this research.

That the test is a measure of competency with the English language is further reflected by the fact that the three lowest scores on this test in the Non-aphasic group are achieved by subjects who are foreign-born, not educated in the United States and with little or no education in their country of birth. But for these three subjects, the difference between the two groups on this test would be even greater.

An analysis of the Eisenson Test data reveals that the Aphasics demonstrate the greatest impairment in the expressive aphasia area. The next area of difficulty is the area of receptive aphasia. The findings of mixed aphasia support those of Weisenburg and McBride, Blatt, and of Eisenson who points out that classification of language difficulties should refer to the predominant areas of disturbance and that "... pure difficulties, either of comprehension of language or of ability to produce language symbols in any form or forms are almost never found."[1] Using Weisenburg and McBride's classification, the Aphasic group in this study fall into the category of *Predominantly Expressive Aphasia.*[2]

The Goldstein-Scheerer Tests. — The Cube and the Stick Tests were developed by Goldstein and Scheerer for the specific purpose of evaluating the intellectual functioning of brain-damaged subjects.

Cube Test. — Tables V (page 62) and VII (page 65), present the mean scores for both groups. As Table IX (page 68), indicates, a t score of 1.79 is not statistically significant at the .05 level of confidence.

An interesting problem, that requires further investigation, is raised as a result of an analysis of the Cube Test data in this research.

Goldstein and Scheerer regard the difficulty with the size of the design, demonstrated by brain-injured subjects on Design I, as an

[1] J. Eisenson, *Examining for Aphasia*, p. 12.
[2] T. Weisenburg and K. E. McBride, *Aphasia*, p. 82.

indication of concrete functioning and an inability to shift to the abstract level of intellectual functioning. Design VI presents a problem, in regard to size similar to Design I, since they are both one-colored designs. In addition, Design VI requires that the subject, for the first time in the test, shift from reproducing the designs on a horizontal plane to making them on an angle.

Many studies have indicated that as a task becomes more complex, the brain-damaged subject tends to exhibit more concrete symptoms, such as perseveration, as well as a tendency to display emotional reactions like lability or what Goldstein refers to as the *catastrophic reaction.* They also demonstrate difficulty in dealing with more than one aspect of the task at a time.

However the indications in this study are that both groups demonstrate less difficulty performing on Design VI than on Design I. While seven aphasics achieve perfect scores on Design I, ten score perfectly on Design VI. In the Non-aphasic group, four receive perfect scores on Design I while five do the same on Design VI.

Since Design I is the first design presented in the Cube Test, many subjects demonstrated such difficulty in the comprehension of the instructions that they failed on the initial presentation of the design. This problem was particularly true for the Aphasic group who, as it has been indicated, demonstrated losses of language ability in the receptive as well as expressive areas on the Eisenson Test for Aphasia. It is possible that some of the *concrete* symptoms exhibited on Design I would not appear if the designs were presented in a different sequence. It is suggested that difficulty exhibited by the Aphasics on this and the other tests may be a result of these receptive losses in language rather than an inability to perform the nonverbal tasks.

Goldstein and Scheerer considered the ability to succeed on the initial step or presentation of a design in the Cube Test a measure of abstract ability. They pointed out further that the inability to profit from the facilitating steps on each design is a definite indication of the impairment of the abstract attitude. They believed that whether or not a patient learns is a reasonable measure of the degree of disturbance in abstract ability.

In this study, all of the aphasic subjects succeed on one or more of the initial presentations of the designs and they all achieve partial scores for succeeding after the presentation of the facilitating steps. Twelve non-aphasics succeed on one or more of the initial steps of the designs and thirteen are able to score after the presentation of the facilitating steps. This data indicates that the loss of abstract ability demonstrated by the brain-damaged subject is not an absolute loss and that these patients are still able to learn. These results support the fiindings of Wepman and Eisenson who did not think there is an absolute loss of the capacity to abstract in brain-damaged patients. Where there is some loss, Eisenson believed, it is not as severe as Goldstein has found, that it tends to occur in patients who are past middle age more often than in younger patients, and that it is more likely an aggravation of a premorbid tendency rather than a new feature of the patient's behavior.

The population in this study are all past middle age. There apparently is some loss of ability to function on an abstract level, as measured by the Cube Test, in both groups. However, the ability of both aphasics and non-aphasics to benefit from the facilitating steps as indicated above seems to support Eisenson's contention that there is not a loss of the abstract attitude but rather a disinclination to assume the abstract attitude.

While there is no statistically significant difference in the level of intellectual functioning between the Aphasic and Non-aphasic groups on this test, there is some indication that the Aphasic group functions on a less concrete or more abstract level than the Non-aphasic group.

The results on this test take on an added significance in view of wide acceptance and high regard this test has achieved as a measure of intellectual functioning. This test was originated by Kohs who presented it as a comprehensive measure of non-verbal intelligence. Wechsler stated that Kohs' enthusiasm for this test was *fully justified.* Speaking of his Block Design subtest which he claims is basically similar to the one employed by Kohs, Wechsler stated that: "The test turns out to be our best single performance item. ... It not only correlates well with total score and individual test items, but is one of the few performance tests that seemingly does measure very much the same sort of thing that verbal tests measure."[3] He concluded that the test is "... an excellent test of general intelligence."[4] In this regard, it should be pointed out that the Aphasic group also demonstrates superiority over the Non-aphasic group on the Block Design test of the Wechsler Bellevue. These results indicate the parallel nature of these two slightly modified versions of the Kohs Block test.

Thurstone[5] and French[6] in separate factor analytic studies reported a *high loading* of the Space Visualization factor in the Cube Test. The results of this study indicate that the Non-aphasic group seems to have suffered a greater loss in this factor than the Aphasic group. However, the difference is not statistically significant.

Stick Copy. — Goldstein and Scheerer pointed out that the apparent simplicity of the task of reproducing purely *geometrical* figures conceals the manner in which the abstract attitude participates in the process of a solution. "Without a generalized *idea* of space in the 'abstract', he would be unable to conceive and hence evolve a purely geometric scheme of direction."[7] The designs on this test, they stated, are simply *configurations of spatial direction.*

The Aphasic group demonstrates superiority over the Non-aphasic group on this test as Tables V (page 62) and VII (page 65) indicate. Table IX (page 68) shows that the difference is significant at the .05 level with a *t* of 2.51.

Bauer and Becka reported similar results in a study employing aphasic and non-aphasic subjects. McFie, *et. al.*, in an investigation of right hemisphere lesion patients without aphasia, conclude that all of the subjects do very poorly in copying simple designs with matchsticks.

Goldstein and Scheerer stated: "... the patient does not con-

[3] D. Wechsler, *Measurement of Adult Intelligence*, p. 92.
[4] *Loc. cit.*
[5] L. L. Thurstone, *A Factorial Study of Perception.*
[6] J. W. French, *The Description of Aptitude and Achievement Tests in Rotated Factors.*
[7] Goldstein and Scheerer, *Abstract and Concrete Behavior: An Experimental Study with Special Tests*, p. 133.

ceive of positional relationship because that meaning is no longer within his grasp."[8] The results of this investigation raise a question as to whether this loss of positional relationship is as absolute as the statement implies. The indications are that the losses are relative and that the Non-aphasics exhibit a significantly greater loss than the Aphasics.

A manifestation of concrete functioning that is typical of brain-damaged patients and seldom observed in normals, according to Goldstein and Scheerer, is the tendency to build the stick pattern very close to the sample figure. Both groups in this study demonstrate this tendency to an equal degree with ten Aphasics and ten Non-aphasics exhibiting this difficulty. This behavior may be a reflection of the subjects' anxiety and uncertainty in a demanding situation and may be a security-getting device. When it is made clear to a subject that he is to make the figure away from the model, he usually is able to do it.

In view of the difficulty the Non-aphasics demonstrate on all of the performance tests, a question may be raised as to whether or not the poor performance is due to some deficit in visual perception. An analysis of the Eisenson test data reveals, however, that none of the Non-aphasics exhibit any loss on the *Visual Agnosia* section. This indicates an ability to recognize configurations visually perceived and seems to rule out visual deficit as a possible cause. Inasmuch as none of the Non-aphasics demonstrate any loss in the area of *Non-verbal Apraxia* on the Eisenson Test, it is unlikely that their difficulty on the non-verbal performance tests is related to any inability to use tools that are part of the body, like the hand, or tools outside the body, such as a pencil. From this analysis, it seems more likely that the difficulty demonstrated by the Non-aphasics on the performance tests stems from some disability in the area of interpretation, and or reproduction of the visual configuration.

The Wechsler Bellevue Intelligence Scale Form I (Performance Section). — The Aphasic group tends to perform somewhat better

[8] *Ibid.*, p. 143.

than the Non-aphasic group on this test as Tables V (page 62) and VII (page 65) show. However, a t of .54 as revealed by Table IX (page 68) is not significant at the .05 level of confidence. Of all the test results, this reflects the smallest difference between the two groups. These results support the findings of Reitan who reported on two pertinent studies. In one study, he used the Wechsler Bellevue Intelligence Scale Form I and in the other, Wechsler's Mental Ability Scale which is quite similar to the first test. In both researches, the left-hemisphere lesion subjects performed better than the right-hemisphere lesion patients on all the performance subtests but none of the differences was significant.

The Picture Arrangement and Digit Symbol subtests require the greatest amount of verbal instruction of all the subtests in the performance section. The Digit Symbol subtest employs numbers and symbols that are similar to letters. This presents a problem for a subject, who like the aphasic, has lost some of his ability in the language area. The aphasics had serious difficulty in understanding the instructions and performed most poorly on these subtests. Since these are timed tests, it was not unusual for much of the time to have expired before the subject would start working. This was particularly true for the Digit Symbol subtest which presented an additional handicap to the left-hemisphere lesion aphasic group. Wechsler pointed out that even normal older subjects are penalized in this test because of the difficulty in motor set and motor speed. In the population under investigation, this problem is enhanced. Since all of the subjects are right-handed, those patients who are paralyzed on the right side are placed in a markedly disadvantageous position on this test.

Cohen, in a factor analytical study, found all five subtests of the Performance section of this test, measured closure in the brain-damaged population. He referred to this factor as non-verbal organization. A second order factor that was *strongly operative* in the test as a whole was "present general intellectual functioning".[9]

[9] J. Cohen, "A Factor-Analytically Based Rationale for the Wechsler Bellevue".

Birren[10] tested a normal population ranging in age from 60 to 74. He, also, found that *closure* was the factor common to all the subtests of the Performance section on this test. He concluded that the individual differences in scores are determined by the individual differences in *stored information* of the subjects.

The results of the present study indicate that while the Aphasic group demonstrates some superiority over the Non-aphasic group in this measure of closure, the difference is not statistically significant. Also that in the non-verbal perceptual area, there is no significant difference in present general intellectual functioning between the two groups.

The Bender Visual Motor Gestalt Test. — This test is commonly included in any test battery but particularly when examining brain-damaged subjects. The test is the only paper and pencil test in the battery employed in this research. Like the Goldstein-Scheerer Stick Test, this test involves spatial orientation in the copying of geometric forms. It differs from the Stick Test in that the forms are not single configurations but a patterning of forms into one gestalt. This demands the additional ability for closure. Studies have indicated that as the task becomes more complex, the brain-damaged subject has more difficulty in assuming the abstract attitude. For this reason, the Bender was included in the present study. The results indicate that brain-damaged subjects have more difficulty with this test than the Stick Test and that the Non-aphasic group has more difficulty than the Aphasic group.

Tables V (page 62) and VII (page 65) present the mean scores on this test and reveal the marked superiority of the Aphasic group over the Non-aphasic group. As Table IX (page 68) shows, a t of 3.58 is significant beyond the .05 level and indicates a much greater difference between the two groups on this test than is demonstrated on the Stick Copy Test.

The Aphasic group demonstrates superiority over the Non-aphasic group on most of the scoring criteria. Table IV (page 57)

[10] J. E. Birren, "A Factorial Analyses of the Wechsler-Bellevue Scale Given to an Elderly Population".

presents the scoring criteria. The difficulty the Non-aphasic group has with spatial orientation on this test is most clearly demonstrated by the greater number of serious errors (i.e., those that receive 8 points) they commit. The Non-aphasics are more likely to distort or rotate the figures than the Aphasics. They also exhibit much greater difficulty in planning the placement of the figures on the paper and tend to place them on the paper without any regard for sequence.

These findings do not support Bender's who reported; "Thus, in a general way, we may conclude that the area most probably involved in disturbances of the visual motor gestalt function, as exemplified by these copied forms, is that between the temporal, parietal and occipital lobes of the dominant hemisphere."[11] In this position Pascal and Suttell are in agreement with Bender.

However, Bauer and Becka[12] reported results similar to those obtained in this study. They employed a population similar to the one used in this study in that the subjects had suffered brain damage as a result of a cerebrovascular accident.

Using the Bender Gestalt Test, Hirschenfang compared a group of right hemiplegic adult patients with cerebral lesions in the dominant hemisphere to a group of left hemiplegic adult patients with cerebral lesions in the non-dominant hemisphere. The mean age of these groups is somewhat similar to the mean age of the groups involved in the current research. He concluded that the right hemiplegic group demonstrated statistically significant superiority over the left hemiplegic group on the over-all test.[13]

McFie, *et. al.*,[14] studied a population quite different from the one investigated in this study. The results of their research were similar to the findings of the present study. They reported that their subjects, all of whom were right cerebral hemisphere lesion patients,

[11] L. Bender, *A Visual Motor Gestalt Test and Its Clinical Use*, p. 75.

[12] R. W. Bauer and D. M. Becka, "Intellect after Cerebro-vascular Accident", pp. 379-384.

[13] S. Hirschenfang, "A Comparison of Bender-Gestalt Reproductions of Right and Left Hemiplegic Patients", p. 439.

[14] J. McFie, M. F. Piercy, and O. L. Zangwill, "Visual-Spatial Agnosia Associated with Lesions of the Right Cerebral Hemisphere", pp. 167-189.

had marked difficulty in the copying of simple designs with pencil or matchsticks. They found that the errors in copying arose from an inability of the subject to maintain a consistent viewpoint or frame of reference. They noted that there was a consistent pattern of visual-spatial disability which was correlated with a lesion involving the posterior portions of the right cerebral hemisphere in right-handed individuals. This visual-spatial disability is noted by this investigator for the right hemisphere lesion group on all the performance tests employed in this research.

The problem presented here will be discussed further in the section on Lateralization of Cerebral Function.

Memory

(Goldstein-Scheerer Stick Test, Reproduction Section)

Guilford[15] has pointed out that while memory is an intellectual factor, it is distinct from thinking factors. The Reproduction section of the Stick Test requires, as Goldstein and Scheerer indicate, the ability to assume the abstract attitude. In addition, it requires the ability to recall these, more or less, meaningless figures and reproduce them after they have been removed from sight. Since memory is intimately associated with learning ability, this test is incorporated into the battery as a measure of memory.

Tables V (page 62) and VII (page 65) show that the Aphasic group achieves a higher mean score than the Non-aphasic group on this test. A t of 2.82, as indicated in Table IX (page 68), is statistically significant at the .05 level of confidence.

The results on this test demonstrate that the Aphasic group is significantly superior to the Non-aphasic group in the ability to recall visual-spatial figures. This finding supports the results of other studies. Stark[16] reported in her study with brain-damaged subjects, on paired-associate learning tasks, that the left-hemisphere lesion group was significantly superior to the right-hemisphere

[15] J. P. Guilford, "The Structure of Intellect".

[16] R. Stark, "An Investigation of Unilateral Cerebral Pathology with Equated Verbal and Visual-Spatial Tasks".

lesion group on visual-spatial learning tasks. McFie, *et. al.*,[17] found that in some of their 8 cases of right-hemisphere lesion subjects, the visual-spatial impairmant was associated with a marked disturbance of memory. Bauer and Becka[18] also reported that the left-hemisphere lesion subjects did significantly better than the right hemisphere lesion subjects on a test of visual-motor form reproduction.

Intertest Correlations

For both the Aphasic and Non-aphasic groups, as is indicated on Tables VI (page 63) and VIII (page 65), there is a low but, at the .05 level of confidence, not significant correlation between the Eisenson test of language ability and all the non-verbal performance tests of intellectual functioning.

The Eisenson Test apparently does not measure the same ability that the non-verbal performance tests of intellectual ability measure. The low correlation also seems to indicate that language plays a minor role in the individual's intellectual functioning in non-verbal areas.

Tables VI (page 63) and VIII (page 65) show that there is a significant correlation at the .05 level for the Aphasic and Non-aphasic groups on all the non-verbal performance tests of intellectual functioning. This reflects a marked degree of overlapping among the various performance tests employed in this study and indicates that they seem to be measuring similar abilities. If this is the case, the question may be raised as to whether future studies or examinations of brain-damaged subjects should eliminate some of the tests in this battery in order to avoid duplication.

Flexibility

Eisenson reported that the perseverating tendency is probably the most frequently found characteristic of the behavior of brain-damaged individuals. He stated that rigidity is "... the perseverating

[17] McFie, Piercy, and Zangwill, *op. cit.*
[18] Bauer and Becka, *op. cit.*

tendency influencing the mode of conduct and the intellectual approach to a situation."[19] Goldstein and Scheerer repeatedly stated that while the normal person can *easily overcome* any difficulty encountered in the solution of the Cube or Stick Tests, this is not true for the brain-damaged patient. The brain-lesion individual, according to them, is incapable of adopting the specified abstract attitude required by the tests. The inability to make this *shift in attitude*, Goldstein and Scheerer referred to as rigidity or lack of flexibility "... which is a symptom of concreteness."[20]

The criteria suggested by Goldstein and Scheerer are employed to determine adaptive flexibility in this study. The Flexibility score is the sum total of all the instances of perseveration on the Cube, the Stick Copy, and the Stick Reproduction Tests. Therefore, the higher the score on this variable, the lower the ability demonstrated to shift and the more rigidity exhibited.

Tables V (page 62) and VII (page 65) indicate a higher mean Flexibility score for the Non-aphasic group. However, a t of 1.76 as shown in Table IX (page 68), is not statistically significant at the .05 level of confidence, indicating that there is no significant difference between the two groups on this test.

Belmont and Birch,[21] in a study of rigidity, employed, as subjects, 175 undergraduate students in psychology. They concluded that two sets of influences seem to be operating simultaneously as determiners of behavioral rigidity. These are situational demands and personality trends. These two interact with each other to produce rigid or non-rigid behavior. Consequently, an individual who generally would respond rigidly in a demanding situation, will demonstrate no rigidity when confronted with tasks which fall in areas of high competence. On the other hand, a person who ordinarily demonstrates no rigidity in behavior may do so when the demands of a situation tap areas of particular incompetence or ambiguity for him.

[19] Eisenson, *op. cit.*, p. 8.

[20] Goldstein and Scheerer, *Abstract and Concrete Behavior*; *an Experimental Study with Special Test*, p. 141.

[21] I. Belmont and H. G. Birch, "Personality and Situational Factors in the Production of Rigidity".

The demands of the performance tests used in this study presented varying amounts of ambiguity and difficulty to the subjects. Many of them, particularly the aphasics, had difficulty in the comprehension of what was expected of them. This was demonstrated in various ways. For example, an aphasic, subject #3, had much difficulty in understanding the instructions at the beginning of the Cube Test. After comprehending the demands, she went on to achieve full or partial scores on the first six designs. As the demands of the task became more difficult, however, as on the final six designs, she was less successful, and there was an increase in the perseverative tendency. While on the first six designs, she scored only one point on flexibility, on the last three designs, she scored 11 points on flexibility. On the first six designs, she achieved a score of 39 successes out of a possible 60, while on the last six designs, she only scored 2 successes out of a possible 60 points.

Belmont and Birch's findings offer an explanation for the lack of consistency of flexibility scores for a given subject on the 3 tests employed. As a test becomes more difficult or the demands more ambiguous for an individual, he will tend to become more rigid. They stated that: "The resultant behavior will be more 'personality dominated' to the extent that the individual feels threatened or in ambiguous circumstances and lacks the skills necessary to respond to the specific situation."[22]

In this regard, they noted that the better adjusted individual tends to perform non-rigidly.

Regardless of whether rigidity is a result of brain-damage as Goldstein contended or an exacerbation of a premorbid personality trait, as Eisenson stated, it apparently plays an important role in the present intellectual functioning of the brain-damaged patient as the results of this study indicates. Some support for Eisenson's explanation may be found in Belmont and Birch's report. Of the 162 subjects who completed all four tasks in their study, 131 demonstrated rigidity on one or more of the tasks while only 31 exhibited no rigidity on the tests. This gives some indication of the prevalence of rigidity personality traits in the non-brain-damaged population.

[22] Belmont and Birch, *op. cit.*

It is likely that the anxiety, uncertainty, and lowered self-concept induced by a brain lesion could make for an "aggravation of a premorbid tendency".[23] toward rigidity. As a result, rigidity becomes a prominent characteristic of brain-damaged individuals.

BRAIN DAMAGE AND INTELLIGENCE

On all of the performance tests employed in this study, both the Aphasic and Non-aphasic groups demonstrate losses. While there is a consistent pattern for the Non-aphasic group to show greater losses than the Aphasic group on all these tests, there is no consistency as to the degree of the losses. The greatest loss that the Non-aphasic group demonstrates as compared to the Aphasic group is in the area of spatial orientation. This is followed by memory for visual-spatial forms. The third area of difficulty is space visualization. The area exhibiting the least degree of loss is closure.

These findings are not consistent with the conclusions of Marie,[24] Goldstein,[25] and Williams[26] who reported that brain injury results in a *general* deficit in intellectual functioning. The differential losses demonstrated by these results tend to support the position taken by Hughlings Jackson,[27] Head,[28] and Weisenburg and McBride,[29] that brain damage makes for a selective type of intellectual impairment rather than a general intellectual deficit.

The question should be raised as to how much of the demonstrated loss of intellectual ability, in both groups, as measured by performance tests is due to brain damage, or age, or other factors.

Wechsler reported that "... most abilities tapped by performance tests decline much more rapidly with age than those involved in

[23] J. Eisenson, *op. cit.*

[24] Marie, as reported in T. Weisenburg and K. McBride, *Aphasia*, pp. 20-24.

[25] K. Goldstein, *After Effects of Brain Injuries in War.*

[26] H. L. Williams, A. Lubin, C. F. Geiselking, "Direct Measurement of Cognitive Deficit: I, Brain Injured Patients".

[27] J. Hughling Jackson, *Selected Writings of J. Hughling Jackson.*

[28] H. Head, *Aphasia and Kindred Disorders of Speech.*

[29] T. Weisenburg and K. McBride, *op. cit.*

verbal tests."[30] He found that intellectual ability begins a fairly constant decline about the age of 25 to 30. This decline is more or less linear between the ages of 30 to 60.

There have been studies that report findings supporting this position. A recent study by Stark (1961) showed a significant correlation between age and visual-motor scores for a group of right-hemisphere lesion subjects, a group of left-hemisphere lesion subjects and a control group of normals. Stark concluded that visual-spatial functioning is more easily disrupted by both age and cerebral pathology than is verbal functioning and that "... an increase in visual-spatial errors with age may also be expected in a normal population."[31]

Studies by Linn and Stern,[32] Chenven, [33]Blackman[34] as well as others have indicated the interfering influence of psychological factors on the behavior of brain-damaged subjects. Wechsler, also, reported that psychoses and psychoneuroses as well as organic brain disease tends to impair functioning on performance tests much more than on verbal tests. Our analysis of the data in this study indicates that there is more than a little evidence of the disabling effect of anxiety and insecurity on the performance of these tasks. It seems apparent that these emotional factors play a part in lowering the scores of subjects in both groups.

Several investigations of brain-damaged patients in which normal control groups were employed, reported no significant differences between the control group and the brain injured groups in certain specified areas of intellectual functioning and significant differences in other specified areas. Stark[35] reported no significant difference between the normal control group and the right-hemisphere lesion group in verbal learning and retention, but the latter group demonstrated significant inferiority to the normal control group in visual-

[30] D. Wechsler, *op. cit.* ,p. 64.
[31] R. Stark, *op. cit.*, p. 286.
[32] L. Linn and M. Stern, "Sodium Amytal in Treatment of Aphasia".
[33] H. Chenven, *Effects of Group Therapy Upon Language Recovery in Predominantly Expressive Aphasia.*
[34] N. Blackman, "Group Psychotherapy with Aphasics".
[35] R. Stark, *op. cit.*

spatial learning and retention. On the other hand, the left-hemisphere lesion group demonstrated no significant difference from the normal control group in ability to learn and retain visual-spatial designs, but was significantly inferior to the normal control group in verbal learning and retention. Here, too, in comparing brain-damaged individuals with normal controls, we find the selective nature of intellectual losses resulting from brain damage. The findings, also, raise the question of the lateralization of cerebral functions which will be discussed in the next section.

LATERALIZATION OF CEREBRAL FUNCTION

The question of lateralization of function takes on added significance as a result of the population in this study separating itself into two distinct groups. In the Aphasic group all are right hemiplegics indicating a cerebral lesion in the left hemisphere and in the Non-aphasic group are all left hemiplegics indicating a lesion in the right cerebral hemisphere.

That aphasia is more likely to occur as a result of a lesion in the left cerebral hemisphere is frequently reported in the literature. Penfield and Roberts'[36] findings are not atypical. Of 175 cases with left cerebral lesions, 128 resulted in aphasia, while of 211 cases with right cerebral lesions, only two exhibited aphasia. In view of the nature of the distribution of the population under investigation, the evidence supports the belief that the left cerebral hemisphere is dominant for language. Is it possible that this dominance for language exhibited by the left hemisphere may be paralleled by a specialization or dominance for visual-spatial relationships by the right hemisphere?

In the present study, the Non-aphasic group consistently scored lower than the Aphasic group on all of the six measured non-verbal criteria, as Table IX (page 68) indicates. These findings are similar to the results reported by Bauer and Becka, Reitan, Anderson, and Stark.

McFie, *et. al.*, found such a marked impairment of visual-spatial

[36] W. Penfield and L. Roberts, *Speech and Brain Mechanisms*.

relationships in their group of right-hemisphere lesion patients, that they concluded: "This might suggest that there is a certain 'division of labor' between the two hemispheres in regard to visual-spatial organization."[37]

Bauer and Wepman found the left hemisphere involved in symbolic language behavior in practically all their subjects, but that non-language intellectual functioning is particularly impaired with right hemisphere lesions. Reitan, Anderson, and Stark came to similar conclusions.

In all of the studies cited, there are marked variations in the nature of the population studied, in the etiology of the brain injury, in the duration of the disability, and in the types of tests administered. Yet, the findings and conclusions of the investigations are very similar. The weight of this accumulation of evidence speaks strongly for making a more specific association between visual-spatial ability and the right hemisphere.

Handedness

Since all the patients in this study are right-handed, the question of the relationship between handedness and cerebral dominance need not be considered. However, it should be indicated that studies by Humphrey and Zangwill, Bauer and Wepman, and Penfield and Roberts questioned the concept of a relationship between handedness and cerebral dominance. They found that the left hemisphere is usually dominant for speech, regardless of handedness. They all reported difficulty in determining pure left-handedness as distinguished from ambidexterity. They concluded that cerebral dominance either does not occur in the so-called left-handed subjects, or tends to be less well developed than in right-handed subjects.

LANGUAGE AND THOUGHT

The Non-aphasic group consistently scores lower than the Aphasic

[37] McFie, Piercy, and Zangwill, *op. cit.*

group on all of the six measured non-verbal criteria, as Table IX (page 68) indicates. On three of these criteria the differences between the two groups are statistically significant. However, on the language test, the Non-aphasic group demonstrates significant superiority over the Aphasic group. There are no consistent relationships between the scores on the language test and those on the performance tests for either group. Although these are extreme cases, they clearly demonstrate the inconsistency of the scores. Subject #5 received the highest score on the language test in the Aphasic Group. He scored the lowest in the group, on the Bender Gestalt Test, the Cube Test, and near the lowest on the other tests. Subject #30 received the lowest score on the language test in the Non-aphasic group. He ranked fourth from the highest score on the Cube, Stick Copy, and Stick Reproduction Tests and slightly lower on the other tests.

These findings are similar to and confirm the results reported by Bauer and Becka, Reitan, Anderson, and Stark. In all these studies, the Non-aphasic group demonstrated superiority over the Aphasic group in verbal skills and inferiority in non-verbal or visual-spatial performance skills.

Goldstein's conclusion that Aphasics or patients with lesions of the left cerebral hemisphere demonstrated a greater impairment of the ability to abstract than other brain damaged subjects is not confirmed by the results of this investigation.

Watson's identification of language and thought as inseparable units that always operate together is not supported by the findings of the present study.

In view of the data, a more tenable position is that of Kennedy and Wolf, Jackson, or Head. They contended that there is a distinction between language and thought and that all the processes of thinking may remain intact even though speech has become defective.

As was pointed out in the discussion on intertest correlation, the lack of any significant correlation between the language test and any of the performance tests of intellectual functioning not only indicates that the tests are measuring different traits but that language seems to play a minor role in the subjects non-verbal intellectual functioning.

While the Aphasic group demonstrates, as Table IX (page 68) shows, significant superiority over the Non-aphasic group on the Stick Tests and the Bender Gestalt Test, on the Wechsler Bellevue Intelligence Scale Form I, (Performance Section) and the Goldstein-Scheerer Cube Test, the superiority is not significant at the .05 level of confidence. If these last two tests measure general intelligence, as was indicated previously, there is no significant difference in the present level of intellectual functioning between the Aphasic and Non-aphasic groups. The indications are that there is no relationship between language and non-verbal intellectual functioning and that the loss of language resulting from the brain injury does not make for a greater impairment of intellectual functioning in non-verbal areas.

LIMITATIONS OF THE STUDY

Tests

The need to conform to a rigid set of instructions in the administration of these tests to a brain-damaged population presented a serious limitation. It was quite apparent during the course of this research that a subject often would not understand what was demanded of him despite the repetition of the instructions. The writer believes that much of the difficulty demonstrated by the subjects on Design I of the Cube Test, as well as in other areas, was due to a lack of understanding of what was required of them rather than due to a defect in the ability to assume the abstract attitude. That this problem exists is indicated in the few instances referred to previously in the section headed Flexibility. In the last two instances mentioned there, the examiner deviated slightly from the prescribed instructions and the subjects were then able to comprehend what was expected of them, and they performed the task successfully. It should be noted that these deviations were rather minimal. In the first instance, it merely involved indicating to the subject that the stick was to be placed on the table and not held in his hand. In the other instance, the examiner demonstrated that the sticks were to be placed together to form something, rather than describing this process by the use of words.

Goldstein and Scheerer recognized this problem and emphasized that: "The instructions given should not 'tie' the examiner in the same way as in the usual standardized tests."[38] They recommend that the examiner should feel free to vary the experimental procedure.

The researcher has come to a similar conclusion. The standardized tests are based upon a normal population. When a subject is examined with the intention of comparing him with the general population, it is important to conform to the same conditions and instructions under which the test was standardized. However, it is doubtful whether this should be the intention when a brain-damaged subject is being evaluated. In such an instance, the intention should be to determine as closely as possible the remaining potential capacity of the patient. From a prognostic point of view in rehabilitation, it would seem to be more important to determine his abilities, not in relation to normals but in relation to other brain-damaged patients. In such an event, the restrictions of standardized instructions for the administration of tests has little meaning. Shontz in his study of the intellectual potential of hemiplegic patients, concluded: "How well a hemiplegic performs in rehabilitation, for example, may be more closely determined by his abilities relative to other hemiplegics than by his abilities relative to to the general population."[39]

Population

During the selection process, the population separated itself into two distinct groups, one group of Aphasics with right hemiplegia, and a group of Non-aphasics with left hemiplegia.

[38] Goldstein and Scheerer, *op. cit.*, p. 30.

[39] F. C. Shontz, "Evaluation of Intellectual Potential in Hemiplegic Individuals", p. 267.

As has been indicated, many authorities found that the loss of language that is commonly associated with left-hemisphere lesions, does not make for a loss of general intelligence. McFie, *et. al.*, reported that in their population of right-hemisphere lesion patients, there is no general loss of abstract ability, as defined by Goldstein, related to the observed visual-spatial defect. The results of the present investigation indicate that there is no significant difference in general intelligence between the left-hemisphere lesion group and the right-hemisphere lesion group. However, it is apparent that the left-hemisphere group is more deficient in language ability and the right-hemisphere group demonstrates a greater deficit in the visual-spatial area.

This raises a question as to how much of the difference in behavior demonstrated on these tests is related to language or to intelligence and how much is related to the locus of the lesion.

Implications

The implications of the findings in this research support the position that language and thought are not necessarily related and that one can think without the use of words.

The evidence raises the question of lateralization of cerebral functioning. The left cerebral hemisphere appears to be dominant for language functions. However, the right cerebral hemisphere seems to be dominant in the visual-spatial area. One may ask whether the tests commonly employed in the evaluation of intelligence of brain-damaged subjects are appropriate and valid. If a test of language ability is an inappropriate measure of the intellectual ability of aphasic subjects, it may be that a non-verbal performance test involving visual-spatial ability is an inappropriate test for right-hemisphere lesion subjects.

In the area of testing, the implications of the results indicate that standardized instructions tend to interfere with obtaining an evaluation of the maximum functioning capacity of brain-injured subjects.

The implications of the data for rehabilitation are significant.

It suggests that a reevaluation be undertaken of the approach employed toward brain-damaged subjects by the therapists from the various disciplines that make up the rehabilitation team. An approach that takes into account the differences revealed in this study between the two groups might make for greater improvement in rehabilitation by the subjects.

6. SUMMARY, CONCLUSIONS, AND RECOMMENDATIONS

SUMMARY

The purpose of this investigation was to determine and evaluate the effect of language disturbance on intellectual functioning among brain-damaged subjects. The population of the study consisted of 30 adult male and female patients between the ages of 52 and 67 years. They were divided into two groups of 15 patients each. One group was diagnosed on admission to the hospital as cerebrovascular accident resulting in hemiplegia *with aphasia* and the other group was diagnosed on admission as cerebrovascular accident resulting in hemiplegia *without aphasia*. None of the subjects had a medical record of more than one cerebrovascular accident. All of the patients were able to ambulate or be transported by wheelchair and were capable of, and agreeable to, participating in this research. They all had been able to understand English premorbidly and were indigent residents of New York City. All but 3 of the subjects were in-patients of the Bird S. Coler Hospital and Home and the remaining 3 subjects were in-patients in the Bellevue Hospital rehabilitation wards. Both of these installations are New York City hospitals under the supervision and control of the New York City Department of Hospitals. All of the patients in the wards who met the delimitations of the study were accepted.

The two groups were equated for age, sex, duration of disability, socio-economic and educational background. There were no significant differences between the groups in any of these areas.

A battery of one language test and 4 non-verbal performance tests of intellectual functioning was administered to each subject. The Eisenson Test was employed to evaluate the level of language ability for both groups. The Goldstein-Scheerer Cube Test, while a good measure of *general intelligence*, was used also to evaluate the intellectual factor of Space Visualization. The Goldstein-Scheerer Stick Test (Copy Section) was employed to measure ability in the area of Spatial Orientation, and the Reproduction Section was used as a measure of Memory. The Wechsler-Bellevue Intelligence Scale Form I (Performance Section), which is also a measure of *present general intellectual functioning* was employed to evaluate the ability for Closure. The Bender Visual Motor Gestalt Test was used to measure ability in tasks involving both Spatial Orientation and Closure. An Adaptive Flexibility score was derived from summing the total of all the perseverations exhibited by the subjects on the Cube Test and the Copy and Reproduction Sections of the Goldstein-Scheerer Stick Test. A summary of the findings based on these tests follows.

Quantitative

1. The mean score of the Aphasic group on the Eisenson Test was 137.33. For the Non-aphasic group, the mean score was 387.33.

A comparison of the scores on the Eisenson Test for the two groups revealed statistically significant differences beyond the .05 level of confidence established for this study. The Non-aphasic group exhibited significant superiority over the Aphasic group.

2. On the Goldstein-Scheerer Cube Test, the mean score for the Aphasic group was 71.43, while for the Non-aphasic group, the mean score was 47.37.

This difference between the two groups was not statistically significant at the .05 level of confidence.

3. The Goldstein-Scheerer Stick Test (Copy Section) revealed a mean score of 145.80 for the Aphasic group and a mean score of 120.73 for the Non-aphasic group.

An analysis of the results on this test revealed that the Aphasic group exhibited superiority over the Non-aphasic group. The difference was statistically significant at the .05 level of confidence.

4. On the Goldstein-Scheerer Stick Test (Reproduction Section),

the Aphasic group mean score was 134.53 and the Non-aphasic mean score was 106.33.

The findings on this test indicated that the Aphasic group performed at a superior level as compared with the Non-aphasic group. The difference was statistically significant at the .05 level of confidence.

5. The mean score of the Aphasic group on the Wechsler-Bellevue Intelligence Scale, Form I (Performance Section) was 38.13. The Non-aphasic group mean score on this test was 33.55.

The results for the test indicated that the difference between the two groups was not statistically significant at the .05 level of confidence.

6. On the Bender Visual Motor Gestalt Test, the Aphasic group mean score was 74.20 and the Non-aphasic group mean score was 138.87.

Since for this test, the higher the score, the poorer the performance, the results revealed that the Aphasic group performed on a superior level to the Non-aphasic group. The difference between both groups was significant statistically beyond the .05 level of confidence.

7. The mean Adaptive Flexibility score for the Aphasic group was 20.93. For the Non-aphasic group, the mean score was 37.40.

For Adaptive Flexibility, a high score reflects a high number of perseverations. This indicates a loss in ability to shift as well as greater rigidity. A comparison of the scores of both groups revealed that the difference between the groups was not statistically significant at the .05 level of confidence.

Qualitative

1. Both groups demonstrated some difficulty in the comprehension of the verbal instructions on all the tests. However, the Aphasic group demonstrated the greatest difficulty with 14 subjects exhibiting this difficulty as compared to 7 Non-aphasics.

2. While none of the Non-aphasics demonstrated lability, 5 Aphasics did. In one case, the testing was halted for the day. In all

the other cases, the symptoms subsided after a short while and the testing was resumed.

3. Nine Non-aphasics overtly expressed anger or hostility toward the examiner, the test, themselves, or others, during the testing. Only 4 Aphasics did the same. However, 7 Aphasics overtly demonstrated marked depression by sighing, crying, or verbalizing it, while only one non-aphasic manifested similar symptoms.

4. Many subjects, in both groups, expressed feelings of inadequacy in one way or another. Although both groups tended to blame themselves for their inability to perform a task, the Non-aphasic group also tended to rationalize the reasons for their failure more often than the Aphasic group.

5. Most subjects, in both groups, demonstrated a high level of aspiration. They exhibited a strong desire and effort to achieve on the tests, as well as to impress the examiner. They were pleased and sometimes elated when they succeeded and were frustrated and depressed by their failures and inadequacies. While some subjects verbalized or indicated a desire to stop when they found a task too difficult, none actually stopped.

6. In some cases, it was quite apparent that emotional and psychological factors played an important part in the difficulty demonstrated on the test performances of both groups.

CONCLUSIONS

The results of this investigation yield the following conclusions regarding the effect of language disturbance on intellectual functioning, for a population of brain-damaged subjects with aphasia and brain-damaged subjects without aphasia.

1. There is no significant relationship between language ability and the ability to perform on a non-verbal intellectual level for a brain-damaged group.

2. The Aphasic group demonstrates statistically significant superiority over the Non-aphasic group in intellectual functioning, in the area of spatial orientation.

3. On tasks involving both spatial orientation and closure the Aphasic group demonstrates statistically significant superiority over the Non-aphasic group.

4. On Memory for visual-spatial figures the Aphasic group demonstrates statistically significant superiority over the Non-aphasic group.

5. While there is a trend indicating that the Aphasic group performs somewhat better on tasks involving general intelligence, the visualization of space, closure and on adaptive flexibility, none of these differences are significantly better than chance.

6. Brain damage makes for a selective type of intellectual impairment rather than a general intellectual deficit.

7. Impairment of language ability is associated with a lesion to the left cerebral hemisphere.

8. Impairment of visual-spatial ability is associated with a lesion to the right cerebral hemisphere.

9. There is no absolute loss of the ability to assume the abstract attitude in brain-damaged subjects.

10. The Non-aphasic group or right cerebral hemisphere-lesion patients, demonstrate a greater loss in ability to assume the abstract attitude than the Aphasic group or left hemisphere-lesion group on non-verbal performance tests of intellectual functioning.

11. More Aphasics than Non-aphasics have difficulty in under-stainding the verbal instructions given on the various tests.

12. Only the aphasic subjects demonstrate lability.

13. More Non-aphasics than Aphasics in the research groups exhibit overt anger or hostility, but more Aphasics than Non-aphasics demonstrate depression.

14. While many subjects in both research groups express feelings of inadequacy, the Non-aphasic group tends to use rationalizations more than the Aphasic group.

15. Most subjects, in both research groups, exhibit a strong desire and effort to achieve on these tests and concern about the approval of the examiner.

TABLE X

Various Test Results for a Group of Fifteen Aphasic Subjects

Subject	Eisenson	Cube	Stick Copy	Stick Reproduction (memory)	Wechsler	Bender	Flexibility		
							Cube	Stick Copy	Stick Reproduction
1	177	120	150	153	62	53	0	1	0
2	112	30	127	89	19	96	21	9	26
3	194	41	151	141	17	97	11	1	4
4	29	34	141	118	20	86	21	4	11
5	298	23	134	124	17	153	9	5	13
6	90	60	155	144	22	58	20	0	3
7	104	104	157	153	52	21	4	0	1
8	192	115	157	153	64	16	0	0	0
9	229	117.5	156	152	70	64	1	1	0
10	98	76	157	151	81	52	15	0	2
11	83	52	151	142	13	50	9	1	5
12	81	32	100	96	4	127	27	17	25
13	175	71	144	144	40	86	9	4	4
14	64	115	154	154	46	80	0	0	0
15	140	81	152	117	45	80	21	1	8
Totals	2066	1071.5	2187	2020	572	1119	168	44	102

TABLE XI

Various Test Results for a Group of Fifteen Non-aphasic Subjects

Subject	Eisenson	Cube	Stick Copy	Stick Reproduction (memory)	Wechsler	Bender	Flexibility		
							Cube	Stick Copy	Stick Reproduction
16	355	0	68	73	7.0	257	31	4	21
17	405	41	140	118	47.5	80	22	2	8
18	392	4	89	93	17.0	217	34	1	8
19	399	103	153	148	75.0	86	6	0	0
20	387	94	114	100	64.0	98	13	21	24
21	399	82	149	127	37.0	111	1	6	2
22	406	46	144	113	55.0	142	28	0	12
23	405	26	111	78	7.0	176	20	11	20
24	395	30	124	90	28.0	90	0	2	3
25	383	101	156	146	50.5	127	0	0	5
26	399	21	117	110	17.0	119	32	14	6
27	350	1	32	32	5.0	246	35	37	44
28	385	11	114	100	13.5	158	28	9	18
29	409	58	155	135	51.0	77	14	0	6
30	341	92	151	132	39.0	100	4	3	6
Totals	5810	710	1810	1595	503.5	2084	268	110	183

RECOMMENDATIONS

The findings in this study raise many questions that merit further investigation.

Is the significantly greater loss in the visual-spatial area that the Non-aphasics demonstrate in this study due to the fact that the lesion is in the right cerebral hemisphere?

To delineate more sharply the role of language ability in intellectual functioning, a study should be undertaken involving subjects who have lesions in the same cerebral hemisphere with half of the subjects demonstrating aphasia and the other half exhibiting no aphasia.

Another problem that calls for greater clarification is a determination, in brain-injured subjects, of how much loss of intellectual ability is due to the brain-damage, to age, or to other factors such as emotional difficulties or basic personality traits.

An investigation should be undertaken to determine the effect that more flexible instructions would have on the test performance of brain-injured subjects.

A determination should be made as to whether non-verbal performance tests of intellectual functioning, involving visual-spatial ability, are valid instruments to determine general intellectual functioning of right cerebral hemisphere-lesion subjects.

Finally, the results of this study indicate that the various members of the rehabilitation team should recognize that many brain-damaged patients, especially Aphasics, may fail on a task because of a lack of comprehension of the instructions. The worker should be quite flexible in his instructions and explanations of a task, employing demonstrations, when they are necessary. In rehabilitation, many tasks require ability in the visual-spatial area. The superior memory and ability for visual-spatial stimuli demonstrated by the aphasic or right hemiplegic patients indicates that they, probably, have greater ability to learn in a rehabilitation program than the non-aphasic or left-hemiplegic patients. However, the primary problem with the aphasic subjects is overcoming the communications difficulty. The non-aphasic or left-hemiplegic patients, because of their difficulty with recall of visual-spatial stimuli, and their lowered ability to perform in the visual-spatial area, require a more simplified, more structured, more repetitive presentation of a visual-motor task in rehabilitation training.

GLOSSARY

As used in this research, certain specific or technical terms are defined as follows:

1. *Adaptive Flexibility* involves the ability to make sudden shifts of organization of a figure, shifts of set or approach to a problem, or shifts of category of responses.[1]

2. *Agnosia* involves the loss of ability to recognize configurations normally received through a given sensory avenue.[2]

3. *Aphasia* is any language problem resulting from organic disturbance of the cortical tissue in which the defect is not due to faulty innervation of the musculature of speech, dysfunction of the peripheral sense organs or general mental deficiency.[3]

4. *Apraxia* refers to the disability in the voluntary use of tools for their intended purpose. The disability may be non-verbal as well as verbal.[4]

5. *Cerebral Vascular Accident* (CVA) refers to a cerebral hemorrhage or thrombosis and often is termed a *stroke*.[5]

6. *Closure* refers to the ability to fuse the perceptual field into a single percept.[6]

7. *Dysphasia* refers to a milder form of language disturbance than implied in aphasia.[7]

8. *Intelligence* is "... the capacity for effective behavior".[8]

[1] J. P. Guilford, "The Structure of Intellect", p. 280.
[2] J. Eisenson, *Examining for Aphasia*, p. 13.
[3] J. P. Wepman, *Recovery from Aphasia*, p. 4.
[4] J. Eisenson, *op. cit.*, pp. 18-19.
[5] J. Gilbert, *Understanding Old Age*, p. 202.
[6] James E. Birren, "A Factorial Analyses of the Wechsler Bellevue Scale Given to an Elderly Population", p. 402.
[7] J. Eisenson, *op. cit.*, p. 1.
[8] Arthur W. Combs, "Intelligence from a Perceptual Point of View", p. 662.

9. *Language* is communication through the use of "... vocal means, written communication, sign communication and gesture".[9]

10. *Memory* involves the ability to learn and to remember things associated, where meaning is of little or no importance.[10]

11. *Space Visualization* involves the ability to perceive spatial patterns accurately and to compare them with each other.[11]

12. *Spatial Orientation* involves the ability to become aware of the spatial order or arrangement of objects perceived visually.[12]

[9] L. M. Dorcas and G. M. Shaffer, *Textbook of Abnormal Psychology*, p. 110.
[10] J. P. Guilford, *op. cit.*, p. 283.
[11] John W. French, *The Description of Aptitude and Achievement Tests in Rotated Factors*, p. 235.
[12] J. P. Guilford, *op. cit.*, p. 271.

BIBLIOGRAPHY

Agranowitz, A., *et. al.*, "Group Therapy as a Method of Retraining Aphasics", *Quarterly Journal of Speech*, 40 (1954), pp. 170-182.

Aita, J. A., S. G. Armitage, R. M. Reitan, and A. Rabinowitz, "The Use of Certain Psychological Tests in the Evaluation of Brain Injury", *Journal of General Psychology*, 37 (1947), pp. 25-44.

Albrecht, Mary, "Suggested Neurological Theory that Justifies Speech Therapy for the Adult Aphasic", *Journal of Rehabilitation*, 28:4 (1962), pp. 20-24.

Allport, Gordon W., "*Personality: A Psychological Interpretation*" (Henry Holt and Co., New York, 1937).

Anderson, A. Lloyd, "The Effect of Laterality Localization of Focal Brain Lesions on the Wechsler-Bellevue Sub-Tests", *Journal of Clinical Psychology*, 7 (1951), pp. 149-153.

Anderson J. O., "Eighteen Cases of Aphasia Studies from the Viewpoint of a Speech Pathologist", *Journal of Speech Disorders*, 10 (1945), pp. 9-33.

——, "*Is* is not the verb for Aphasia", *Journal of Speech Disorders*, 11 (1946), pp. 135-138.

Appelbaum, S. A., "Expanded Word Test as a Measure of Psychological Deficit Associated with Brain Damage", *Journal of Clinical Psychology*, 19:1 (1963), pp. 78-84.

Aronson, M., L. Shatin, and J. C. Cook, "Socio-Psychotherapeutic Approach to the Treatment of Aphasic Patients", *Journal of Speech and Hearing Disorders*, Vol. 21, No. 3 (September, 1956), pp. 352-364.

Backus, O., "Rehabilitation of Aphasia Veterans", *Journal of Speech Disorders*, 10 (1945), pp. 149-153.

——, "The Use of Group Structure in Speech Therapy", *Journal of Speech and Hearing Disorders*, 17 (1952), pp. 116-122.

Bateman, Frederic, *On Aphasia or Loss of Speech and the Localization of the Faculty of Articulate Language* (John Churchill & Sons, London, 1870).

Bauer, R. W. and D. M. Becka, "Intellect after Cerebrovascular Accident", *Journal of Nervous and Mental Diseases*, Vol. 120, No. 5 (Nov.-Dec. 1954), pp. 379-384.

——, and J. M. Wepman, "Lateralization of Cerebral Functions", *Journal of Speech and Hearing Disorders*, Vol. 20, #2 (June 1955), pp. 171-177.

Bay, E., "Present Concepts of Aphasia", *Geriatrics*, 19:5 (1964), pp. 319-331.

Belmont, I. and H. G. Birch, "The Generality and Specificity of Rigidity", *Journal of General Psychology* (1958).

——, "Personality and Situational Factors in the Production of Rigidity", *Journal of General Psychology*, 62 (1960), pp. 3-17.

Bender, Lauretta, *A Visual Motor Gestalt Test and Its Clinical Use* (American Orthopsychiatric Association, Res. Monog. No. 3, 1938).

Bergman, P. and M. Green, "Aphasia: Effect of Intravenous Sodium Amytal", *Neurology*, 1 (1951), pp. 471-475.

Berry, M. F. and J. Eisenson, *The Defective in Speech* (F. S. Crofts and Company, New York, 1942).

Billows, B. W., "Observations of the Use of Sodium Amytal in the Treatment of Aphasia", *Medical Record*, 162, 12 (1949).

Birch, Herbert G., "Perceptual and Sensory Integration in Brain Damage", *Journal of General Psychology*, 105:1 (1964), p. 17.

——, and Ira Belmont, "Functional Levels of Disturbance Manifested by Brian-damaged (Left Hemiplegic) Patients as Revealed in Rorschach Responses", *Journal of Nervous, Mental Diseases*, 132 (1961), pp. 410-416.

——, and Joan Lee, "Cortical Inhibition in Expressive Aphasia", *American Medical Association, Archives of Neurology and Psychiatry*, Vol. 74 (November 1955), pp. 514-517.

Birren, James E., "A Factorial Analyses of the Wechsler-Bellevue Scale Given to an Elderly Population", *Journal of Consulting Psychology*, 16 (1952), pp. 399-405.

Blackman, N., "Group Psychotherapy with Aphasics", *Journal of Nervous and Mental Diseases*, 11 (1950), pp. 154-163.

——, and L. L. Tureen, "*Aphasia:* A Psychosomatic Approach in Rehabilitation", *Transactions of American Neurological Association*, 73 (1948), pp. 193-196.

Blatt, B., *The Problem of Language Localization into Specific Brain Areas*. Ph. D. Dissertation, New York University, 1949.

Boneau, C. A., "The Effects of Violation of Assumptions Underlying the t-test", *Psychological Bulletin*, Vol. 57, No. 1 (January 1960), pp. 43-64.

Boyd, Foster, "A Provisional Quantitative Scoring with Preliminary Norms for the Goldstein-Scheerer Cube Test", *Journal of Clinical Psychology*, 5 (1949), pp. 148-153.

Broca, P., "Location of the Speech Center", translated by J. Kann. *Journal of Speech and Hearing Disorders*, 15 (1950).

Brown, Joe R. and Josephine Simonson, "A Clinical Study of 100 Aphasic Patients; Observations on Lateralization and Localization of Lesions", *Neurology*, 7 (1957), pp. 777-783.

Butfield, E. and O. L. Zangwill, "Re-education in Aphasia; A Review of 70 cases", *Journal of Neurology, Neurosurgery, Psychiatry*, 9 (1946), pp. 75-79.

Chenven, H., *Effects of Group Therapy upon Language Recovery in Predominantly Expressive Aphasic Patients*. Ph.D. Dissertation, New York University, 1953.

Cohen, Jacob, "Factors Underlying Wechsler Bellevue Performance of Three Neuropsychiatric Groups", *Journal of Abnormal and Social Psychology*, No. 47 (1952), pp. 359-365.

——, "A Factor-Analytically Based Rationale for the Wechsler-Bellevue", *Journal of Consulting Psychology*, No. 16 (1952), pp. 272-277.

Cohen, Leon, "Perception of Reversible Figures After Brian Injury", *Archives of Neurology and Psychiatry*, 81 (1959), pp. 765-775.

Colin, Cherry, E., *et. al.*, "Experiments on the Complete Suppression of Stammering", *Nature*, November 5 (1955), p. 874.

Combs, Arthur W., "Intelligence from a Perceptual Point of View", *Journal of Abnormal and Social Psychology*, Vol. 47 (1952), pp. 622-673.

Copi, Irvin M., *The Growth of Concepts In Language, Thought, and Culture*, P. Henle (ed.) (Ann Arbor, Mich. University of Michigan Press, 1958), pp. 25-48.

Curtin, James T., *A Factor Analysis of Verbal and Non-Verbal Tests of Intelligence* (= *The Catholic University of America, Educational Research Monographs*, Feb, 1. 1952, Vol. XVI, No. 4).

Cutsforth, Thomas D., "Personality Crippling Through Physical Diasability", *Journal of Social Issues*, Vol. IV, No. 4 (Fall, 1948), p. 62.

Doehring, Donald G. and R. M. Reitan, "MMPI Performance of Aphasic and Non-aphasic Brain Damaged Patients", *Journal of Clinical Psychology*, 16 (1960), pp. 307-309.

——, R. M. Reitan, and Halligren Klove, "Changes in Patterns of Intelligence Test Performance Associated with Homonymous Visual Field Defects", *Journal of Nervous Mental Diseases*, 132 (1961), pp. 227-233.

Dorcus, R. M. and G. W. Shaffer, *Textbook of Abnormal Psychology* (Williams and Wilkins, Baltimore, 1934).

Edwards, Allen L., *Statistical Methods for the Behavioral Sciences* (Rinehart, New York, 1954).

——, and Richard Auger, "The Effect of Aphasia on the Perception of Precedence", *Proceedings of the 73rd Annual Convention of American Psychological Assn.*, pp. 207-208.

Eisenson, J., *Examining For Aphasia, A. Manual for the Examination of Aphasia and Related Disturbances* (The Psychological Corporation, New York, 1954).

——, "Language and Intellectual Modifications Associated with Right Cerebral Damage", *Language and Speech*, 5:2 (1962), pp. 49-53.

——, "Aphasic Language Modifications as a Disruption of Cultural Verbal Habits", *Journal of American Speech and Hearing Associations*, 5:2 (1963), pp. 503-506.

Franz, S. K., "On Certain Fluctuations in Cerebral Function in Aphasics", *Journal of Experimental Psychology*, 3 (1930), pp. 355-364.

——, *Nervous and Mental Re-education* (New York, MacMillan Company, 1923).

——, "Studies in Re-education: The Aphasias", *Journal of Comparative Psychology*, 4 (1924), pp. 349-429.

——, "The Relations of Aphasia", *Journal of General Psychology*, 3 (1930), pp. 401-411.

French, John W., *The Description of Aptitude and Achievement Tests in Rotated Factors* (University of Chicago Press, Chicago, Ill., 1951).

Freud, Esti D., "Clinical Language Rehabilitation of Veterans; Methods and Results", *Journal of Psychiatry*, 107 (1951), pp. 881-889.

Gilbert, J., *Understanding Old Age* (The Ronald Press, New York, 1952).

Goldhamer, H., "Use of Language in Dreams in Analysis of Aphasic Deficits", *Archives of Neurology and Psychiatry*, 62 (1949), pp. 725-727.

Goldstein, Kurt, *The Organism* (American Book Company, New York, 1939).
——, *After Effects of Brain Injuries in War* (Grune and Stratton, New York, 1942).
——, "The Mental Changes Due to Frontal Lobe Damage", *Journal of Psychology*, 17 (1944), pp. 187-208.
——, *Language and Language Disturbances* (Grune and Stratton, New York, 1948).
—— and M. Scheerer, "Abstract and Concrete Behavior; An Experimental Study with Special Tests", *The American Psychological Association*, Vol. 53, No. 2 (Northwestern University, Evanston, Ill., 1941).
Granick, L., *Aphasia, A Guide to Retraining* (Grune and Stratton, New York, 1947).
Grayson, Morris, Ann Powers and Joseph Levi, *Psychiatric Aspects of Rehabilitation* (The Institute of Physical Medicine and Rehabilitation, New York University-Bellevue Medical Center, 1952).
Guilford, J. P., "The Structure of Intellect", *Psychological Bulletin*, Vol. 53, No. 4 (July 1956), pp. 267-293.
Head, H., "Speech and Cerebral Localization", *Brain*, 46 (1923), pp. 355-528. *Aphasia and Kindred Disorders of Speech* (Macmillan Company, New York, 1926), two volumes.
——, "Hughlings Jackson on Aphasia and Kindred Disorders of Speech", *Brain*, 38 (1915), pp. 1-27.
Hebb, D. O., *The Organization of Behavior* (John Wiley and Sons, Inc., New York, 1949).
Heilbrun, A. B., Jr., "Psychological Test Performance as a Function of Lateral Localization of Cerebral Lesion", *Journal of Comparative Physiological Psychology*, 49 (1956), pp. 10-14.
——, "Lateralization of Cerebral Lesion and Performance on Spatial-temporal Tasks", *Archives of Neurology and Psychiatry*, 1 (1959), pp. 282-287.
——, "An Immediate Memory Modification of the Block Design Task; Relative Performances of Brain-Damaged and Control Subjects", *Journal of Consulting Psychology*, 23 (1959), pp. 390-394.
Helson, Harry, *Theoretical Foundations of Psychology* (D. Van Nostrand Company, Inc., New York, 1951).
Hirschenfang, S., "A Comparison of Wais Scores of Hemiplegic Patients with and without Aphasia", *Journal of Clinical Psychology*, 16 (1960), 351-352.
——, "A Comparison of Bender-Gestalt Reproductions of Right and Left Hemiplegic Patients", *Journal of Clinical Psychology*, 16:4 (1960), p. 439.
Huber, Mary W., "Speech and Vocational Placement", *The Crippled Child*, October 1949, pp. 1-2.
Humphrey, M. E. and O. L. Zangwill, "Re-education in Aphasia; A Review of 70 cases", *Journal of Neurology, Neurosurgery and Psychiatry*, 15 (1952), pp. 184-193.
Hunt, J. Mc V., *Personality and Behavior Disorders* (Ronald Press, New York, 1944), 2 volumes.
Hutt, M., *A Tentative Guide for the Administration and Interpretation of the Bender Gestalt Test* (U.S. Army Adjutant General's School, 1945) (Restricted).

Jackson, J. Hughling, *Selected Writings of J. Hughling Jackson*, J. Taylor (ed.) (Hodder and Stoughton, London, 1931).
Jones, Lyle V. and Joseph M. Wepman, "Dimensions of Language Performance in Aphasia", *Journal of Speech, Hearing Disorders*, 4 (1961), pp. 220-232.
Kennedy, F. and A. Wolf, "The Relationship of Intellect to Speech Defect in Aphasic Patients", *Journal of Nervous and Mental Disease*, 84 (1936), pp. 125-145.
Kennedy, L., "Remedial Procedures for Handling Aphasic Patients", *Archives of Neurology and Psychiatry*, 57 (1942), pp. 646-649.
Lashley, K. F., "Factors Limiting Recovery after Central Nervous Lesions", *Journal of Nervous and Mental Disease*, 88 (1938), p. 741.
Leutenegger, R. R., "A Bibliography on Aphasia", *Journal of Speech and Hearing Disorders*, 16 (1951), pp. 280-292.
Levitt, Herbert, Ronald Sindberg, Bernard Messert and Anita Albaum, "The Laterality Hypothesis in the Assessment of Localized Brain Damage", *Journal of Consulting Psychology*, Vol. 30 (April 1966), No. 2, p. 180.
Liddell, E. G. T. and C. G. Phillips, "Thıesholds of Cortical Representation", *Brain*, Vol. 73, Part 2 (June 1950), pp. 125-140.
Linn, L., "Sodium Amytal in Treatment of Aphasics", *Archives of Neurology and Psychiatry*, 58 (1947), p. 357.
—— and M. Stern, "Sodium Amytal in Treatment of Aphasia", *Bulletin United States Army Medical Department*, 5 (1946).
Loranger, Armand W., and Henryk Musiak, "The Performance of Aged Females on Five Non-language Tests of Intellectual Functions", *Journal of Clinical Psychology*, 16 (1960), pp. 189-191.
Mairov, F. F. and F. Z. Pau, "Evolutionary Physiological Investigation of Motor Disorders of Speech in Cases of Cranial-Brain Traumata", *Zh. Vyssh. Nervn. Deiatel*, 2 (1951), pp. 654-659.
Marie, Pierre, "Revision de la Question de l'Aphasie", *Semaine Med*, 1906.
Marks, S., M. Taylor and H. Rusk, "Rehabilitation of the Aphasic Patient", *Neurology*, 7 (1957), pp. 837-843.
McFie, J., M. F. Piercy, and O. L. Zangwill, "Visual-Spatial Agnosia Associated with Lesions of the Right Cerebral Hemisphere", *Brain*, 73 (1950), pp. 167-189.
Menninger, William C., "Emotional Adjustments for the Handicapped", *The Crippled Child*, December 1949, p. 1.
Meyers, R., "Aphasia, A Problem in Differential Diagnosis and Reeducation", *Quarterly Journal of Speech*, 33 (1937), pp. 357-377.
Meyers, R., "Relation of 'Thinking' and Language: An Experimental Approach using Dysphasic Patients", *Archives of Neurology and Psychiatry*, 60, 119 (1948), p. 112.
Mills, Charles K., "Treatment of Aphasia by Training", *Journal of the American Medical Association*, XLIII, (May 1904), pp. 1940-1949.
Moran, Louis, J. McGaughron, S. Laurence, and Don Leventhal, "Intra-individual consistency in conceptualization", *Journal Abnormal, Social Psychology*, 55 (1957), pp. 194-196.
Müller, Max, *The Science of Thought* (New York, 1887), two volumes.
Nadel, A. B., "A Quantitative Analysis of Behavior Following Cerebral

Lesions", *Archives of Psychology* (New York, 1938), No. 224.

Nielson, J. M., *Agnosia, Apraxia, Aphasia*, 2nd Edition (Paul Hoeber Company, New York, 1946).

——, "Aphasia Rehabilitation: A Report of 9 Successful Cases", *Military Surgeon*, 14 (1954), pp. 462-469.

Office of Defense Mobilization, "Summary-Report of the Task Force on the Handicapped", *Journal of Rehabilitation*. March-April 1952, p. 4.

Parsons, Oscar A., *et. al.*, "Impairment of Abstracting Ability in Multiple Sclerosis", *Journal of Nervous, Mental Disorders*, 125 (1957), pp. 221-225.

Pascal, G., "Simple Methods for the Objective Determination of Some Effects of Electro-convulsive Therapy on the Individual Patient", *Journal of Abnormal and Social Psychology*, 1951.

——, and Barbara Suttel, *The Bender Gestalt Test* (Grune and Stratton, New York, 1951).

Penfield, W. and T. Rassmussen, *The Cerebral Cortex of Man: A Clinical Study of Localization of Function* (Macmillan Company, New York, 1950).

——, and L. Roberts, *Speech and Brain Mechanism* (Princeton University Press, Princeton, N. J., 1959).

Reinbold, M., "Some Aspects of Human Orientation in Space", *Brain*, Vol. 76, Part 3 (Sept. 1953), pp. 337-363.

"Rehabilitation of the Hemiplegic" (edited by Medical Division of Sharpe and Dohme, Inc., Pennsylvania, No. 14, 1952).

Reitan, Ralph M., "Intellectual Function in Aphasic and Non-aphasic Brain-injured Subjects", *Neurology*, Vol. 3, No. 3 (Minneapolis, March, 1953), pp. 202-212.

——, "Intelligence and Language Functions in Dysphasic Patients", *Diseases of the Nervous System*, Vol. XV, No. 5 (May 1954), pp. 2-8.

——, "Certain Differential Effects of Left and Right Cerebral Lesions in Human Adults", *Journal of Comparative and Physiological Psychology*, Vol. 48, No. 6 (December, 1955), pp. 474-478.

——, "Qualitative and Quantitative Mental Changes Following Brain Damage", *Journal of Psychology*, 46 (Oct. 1958), pp. 339-346.

——, "Effects of Brain Damage on a Psychomotor Problem-Solving Task", *Perceptual Motor Skills*, 9 (1959), pp. 211-215.

Reitan, R. M. and E. L. Tarsches, "Differential Effects of Lateralized Brain Lesion on the Trail-making Test", *Journal of Nervous and Mental Diseases*, 129 (1959), pp. 257-262.

Revez, G. (ed.), *Thinking and Speaking: A Symposium* (North-Holland Publishing Company, Amsterdam, 1954).

Riklan, Manual and Leonard Diller, "Visual, Motor Performance Before and After Chemosurgery of the Basal Ganglia in Parkinson's", *Journal of Nervous and Mental Diseases*, 132 (1961), pp. 309-314.

Robbins, S. D., "Examining and Re-education of Aphasics", *Journal of Speech Disorders*, 4 (1939), pp. 15-24.

Scargill, M. H., "Modern Linguistics and Recovery from Aphasia", *Journal of Speech and Hearing Disorders*, 19 (1954), pp. 507-513.

Schaffer, G. W. and R. S. Lazarus, *Fundamental Concepts in Clinical Psychology* (McGraw-Hill Book Company, Inc., New York, 1952).

Schiller, F., "Aphasia Studied in Patients with Missile Wounds", *Journal of Neurology, Neurosurgery and Psychiatry*, 10 (1947).

Schuell, H., V. Carrol, B. S. Street, "Auditory Impairment in Aphasia; Significance and Retraining Techniques", *Journal of Speech and Hearing Disorders*, 18 (1953), pp. 14-21.

——, V. Carrol, B. S. Street, "Clinical Treatment of Aphasia", *Journal of Speech and Hearing Disorders*, 20 (1955),

Schuell, H. and James J. Jenkins, "The Nature of Language Deficit in Aphasia", *Psychological Review*, 66 (1959), pp. 45-67.

Sheehan, V. M., "Rehabilitation of Aphasics in an Army Hospital", *Journal of Speech Disorders*, 11 (1946), pp. 149-157.

——, "Techniques in the Management of Aphasics", *Journal Speech and Hearing Disorders*, 13 (1948), pp. 241-246.

Shontz, F. C., "Evaluation of Intellectual Potential in Hemiplegic Individuals", *Journal of Clinical Psychology*, 13 (1957), pp. 267-269.

Singer, D. and A. A. Low, "The Brain in Case of Motor Aphasia in which Improvement Occurred with Training", *Archives of Neurology and Psychiatry*, 29 (1933), pp. 162-165.

Spearman, C., *The Abilities of Man* (The Macmillan Company, New York, 1927).

Stark, R., "An Investigation of Unilateral Cerebral Pathology with Equated Verbal and Visual-Spatial Tasks", *Journal of Abnormal and Social Psychology*, No. 2 (1961), pp. 282-287.

Stephanson, W., "Tetrad-Differences for Verbal Subtests Relative to Nonverbal Subtests", *Journal of Educational Psychology*, 22 (1931), pp. 334-340.

Stivers, C. G., "Re-education in Aphasia", *Journal of American Medical Association*, 81 (1923), pp. 1355, 1356.

Strother, Charles R., *et al.*, "The Relationship Between Advanced Age and Mental Abilities", *Journal of Abnormal Social Psychology*, 55 (1957), p. 202.

Taylor, James B., "The Bender Gestalt as a Measure of Intelligence and Adjustment in the Lower Intellectual Range", *Journal of Consulting Psychology*, December, Vol. 29, No. 6 (1965), p. 595.

Thurstone, L. L., *A Factorial Study of Perception* (Univ. of Chicago Press, Chicago, Ill., 1944).

Travis, L. E., *Speech Pathology* (Appleton, New York, 1931), p. 331.

Ullman, Montague and Gruen, Arno, "Behavioral Changes in Patients with Strokes", *American Journal of Psychiatry*, 117 (1961), pp. 1004-1009.

Vogel, William, "Some Effects of Brain Lesion on MMPI Profiles", *Journal of Consulting Psychology*, 26:5 (1962), pp. 412-415.

Walker, Helen, M. and Joseph Lev, *Elementary Statistical Methods* (Henry Holt, New York, 1958).

Watson, J. B., "Is Thinking Merely the Action of Language Mechanisms", *British Journal of Psychology*, 11 (1920), pp. 87-104.

——, *Behaviorism* (W. W. Norton and Company Inc., New York, 1924).

Wechsler, David, *The Measurement of Adult Intelligence* (The Williams and Wilkins Company, Baltimore, 1949).

Weigl, E., "On the Psychology of So-called Processes of Abstraction", *Journal of Abnormal and Social Psychology*, 36 (1941), pp. 3-33.

Weinstein, S. and H. Teuber, "The Role of Preinjury Education and Intelligence

Level in Intellectual Loss after Brain Injury", *Journal of Comparative, Physiological Psychology*, 50 (1957), pp. 535-539.

Weisenburg, T. and K. E. McBride, *Aphasia* (The Common-Wealth Fund, New York, 1935).

Wepman, J. M., *Recovery from Aphasia* (The Ronald Press Company, New York, 1951).

——, "A Conceptual Model for the Processes Involved in Recovery from Aphasia", *Journal of Speech and Hearing Disorders*, 1953, pp. 4-13.

——, *A Selected Bibliography on Brain Impairment, Aphasia and Organic Psychodiagnosis* (Language Research Associates, Chicago, Ill. 1961).

Werner, Heinz, "Microgenisis and Aphasia", *Journal of Abnormal and Social Psychology*, 52, No. 3 (May 1954), pp. 347-353.

Williams, Al. L., A. Lubin and C. F. Geisiking, "Direct Measurement of Cognitive Deficit: I, Brian Injured Patients", *Journal of Mental Sciences*, 1956.

Wilson, S. A. K., *Aphasia* (Kogin, Parel, Trench, Trubner Company, London, 1926).

Wood, N. E., "A Comparison of Right Hemiplegics with Left Hemiplegics in Visual Perception", *Journal of Clinical Psychology*, 11 (1955), pp. 378-380.

Zangwill, O. L., *Cerebral Dominance and its Relation to Psychological Function* (Oliver and Boyd, 1960, Edinburgh, Scotland).

Zaslow, Robert W., "A Study of Concept Formation in Normals, Mental Defectives and Brain-Damaged Adults", *Genetic Psychology Monograph*, 63 (1961), pp. 279-388.

44. THEODORE M. DRANGE: Sentential Meaninglessness in the Border Area of Linguistics and Philosophy. 1966. 218 pp. Gld. 23.—

45. WARREN H. FAY: Temporal Sequence in the Perception of Speech. 1966. 126 pp., 29 figs. Gld. 19.50

46. A. CAPELL: Studies in Socio-Linguistics. 1966. 167 pp., 2 tables. Gld. 22.—

47. BOWMAN CLARKE: Language and Natural Theology. 1966. 181 pp. Gld. 26.—

51. HOWARD R. POLLIO: The Structural Basis of Word Association Behavior. 1966. 95 pp., 4 folding tables, 8 pp. graphs, figs. Gld. 16.—

54. RANDOLPH QUIRK and JAN SVARTVIK: Investigating Linguistic Acceptability. 1966. 118 pp., 14 figs., 4 tables. Gld. 15.—

56. NOAM CHOMSKY: Topics in the Theory of Generative Grammar. 1966. 95 pp. Gld. 12.—

59. JOSEPH H. GREENBERG: Language Universals, With Special Reference to Feature Hierarchies. 1966. 89 pp. Gld. 18.—

60. CHARLES F. HOCKETT: Language, Mathematics, and Linguistics. 1967. 243 pp., many figs. Gld. 21.—

65. ROGER L. BROWN: Wilhelm von Humboldt's Conception of Linguistic Relativity. 1967. 132 pp. Gld. 16.—

MOUTON · PUBLISHERS · THE HAGUE

Bei Fragen zur Produktsicherheit wenden Sie sich bitte an:
If you have any questions regarding product safety,
please contact:

Walter de Gruyter GmbH
Genthiner Straße 13
10785 Berlin
productsafety@degruyterbrill.com